Endocrine Diseases of the Dog

EDWARD T. SIEGEL, V.M.D., Ph.D.

Late Professor of Medicine
Chief, Endocrine Service
School of Veterinary Medicine
University of Pennsylvania
Philadelphia, Pennsylvania

Lea & Febiger • *1977* • *Philadelphia*

The logo on the front cover is used through the courtesy and with the permission of the American Veterinary Medical Association and the American Diabetes Association.

Library of Congress Cataloging in Publication Data

Siegel, Edward T
Endocrine diseases of the dog.

Includes bibliographies and index.
1. Dogs—Diseases. 2. Veterinary endocrinology.
I. Title [DNLM: 1. Dog diseases. 2. Endocrine diseases—Veterinary. SF992.E5 S571e]
SF992.E53S53 636.7′08′964 76-56826
ISBN 0-8121-0570-2

Library of Congress Catalog Card Number

PRINTED IN THE UNITED STATES OF AMERICA

Print Number: 3 2 1

This book is dedicated to my wife Harriet
for her support and encouragement
and to my children Jonathan, Aaron and Rachel

Preface

Veterinary endocrinology is still in the embryologic state of development, and its growth is hampered by the limited number of individuals trained in the discipline. A need exists for trained investigators to develop a critical body of knowledge on the basic endocrinology and clinical endocrinology of the dog. Over the years I have accumulated many authors' findings of important endocrinologic data about the dog. This large body of information became available because basic endocrinologic research was done with the dog as the animal model. Regrettably, the literature is still incomplete.

In correlating what is known about endocrine diseases in the dog, I have drawn information from many sources, and *basic* discussions of the abnormalities represent compilations of data from the veterinary and medical literature. However, details pertaining to many of the *clinical* endocrinopathies are based on my experience. This book is not a detailed and complete textbook for the trained endocrinologist; rather it is directed to the student of veterinary medicine and the veterinary practitioner who graduated a number of years ago, when veterinary endocrinology was not so advanced as it is today.

So that the reader would not find this study laborious, I have provided documentation sparingly, and only when I have deemed it absolutely necessary. Wherever a controversial point appeared in the literature, I have tried to present each side of the particular argument, attempting, with difficulty, to remain unbiased. I would remind the reader that a book naturally represents the author's interpretation of available facts.

I have attempted to discuss the anatomy, histology, physiology, pathologic physiology, prognosis, and treatment in a logical sequence in most chapters. This format was chosen to make the book more readable.

Finally, I have tried to be selective rather than all inclusive when listing the references. At the end of each chapter is a list of *Selected Reading.* This bibliography is intended to give the reader the basic information he needs as well as the understanding to expand his background on the information presented. It is not intended as an extensive bibliography, as might be expected in the standard textbook.

I would like to thank Mr. Christian C. F. Spahr, Jr., of Lea & Febiger for his interest and encouragement in the preparation of this book; Dr. John T. McGrath for his contribution of many gross and microscopic photographs of the different pathologic abnormalities; Rose Mazur for her help in preparing this manuscript; and Dr. Nancy Leveque for her help in proofreading this manuscript.

Philadelphia, Pennsylvania EDWARD T. SIEGEL

Contents

Chapter 1
Introduction

The endocrine system is composed of glands that utilize vascular channels for dispersion of their secretions. The word endocrine (*endo*, within + *krinein*, to separate) implies *internal secretion,* in contrast with exocrine glands, which excrete externally onto the surfaces of the body or through its passages to the outside. Glands of external secretion transport their products via ducts, whereas glands of internal secretion (endocrine) are ductless.

The substances secreted by the endocrine glands are called hormones; they are chemical messengers. Hormones are produced in a specific endocrine tissue, and are diffused or transported via the blood or lymph to other parts of the body where they modify activity in such a way as to affect homeostasis. These endocrine glands themselves comprise the pituitary (the adenohypophysis and neurohypophysis), thyroid, parathyroid, adrenal cortex and medulla, islets of Langerhans of the pancreas, ovary, testis, placenta, and pineal gland.

Clinical endocrinology is the study of diseases of the endocrine glands — diseases that result either from an insufficiency or from an excess of specific hormones. An insufficiency of a particular hormone may not always be attributable to a decreased secretion of that hormone. The condition may also exist when the amount of hormone secreted is normal, but its excessive binding by plasma proteins decreases the availability of the free hormone at the target tissue. This latter type of abnormality is seen in certain cases of hypothyroidism in which thyroxine is secreted in normal amounts, but its binding in the plasma is increased. An insufficiency can also occur if there is increased catabolism or destruction of the hormone produced. Under these circumstances also, the specific hormone is being secreted in normal amounts. The increased turnover of the hormone results in a decreased level in the circulation for its effect. Finally, an insufficiency may be the result of an abnormal response of the target tissue. In this case the circulating level of the hormone is normal, but the defect in the target tissue produces a less-than-normal response. An example of this type of abnormality is nephrogenic diabetes insipidus, in which antidiuretic hormone (ADH) is secreted in normal amounts. The defect is an abnormality in the kidney tubule, which decreases its response to ADH.

MECHANISM OF HORMONE ACTION

The precise way in which some hormones act on the cell is not known. Some actions of hormones appear to be quite complex, whereas the mechanism of others seems to be relatively simple. Hormones may act by affecting the transport of various substances through the membrane of cells; or they may modify the amount of activity or production of certain enzymes or specific proteins. In addition, hormones may alter the availability of cofactors or act as coenzymes themselves. Additionally, it has been shown that hormones may stimulate or inhibit the formation of a hormonal mediator.

Although hormones do not themselves initiate reactions in the body, they do influence the rate at which certain physiologic events proceed. If a hormone is completely absent, its specific action will, in most instances, continue to exist, but at a rate far less than normal. Hormones have functions that are in many ways similar to those of catalysts. Most hormonal actions are directly related to the amount of the hormone present, at least within a certain physiologic range. The greater the amount of hormone present, the greater is the response. However, there are limits to this physiologic phenomenon.

TRANSPORT, METABOLISM, AND EXCRETION OF HORMONES

Normally hormones are secreted by endocrine tissues. However, all hormones are not water-soluble and thus are negligibly available in the free form in plasma at physiologic levels. The binding of hormones to plasma proteins produces a transport mechanism that allows an increased amount of the hormone to be carried in the plasma. This hormone-protein transport system is in equilibrium with the smaller amount of the hormone in the free state. An example of this type of mechanism occurs with thyroxine, which is bound to specific plasma proteins. A similar transport system is known for a number of the steroidal hormones, both the corticosteroids and the gonadal steroids. In other instances the hormone itself, being water-soluble, is in its free or unbound form in the plasma.

The metabolism of hormones usually is carried out in peripheral tissues. In some instances a specific tissue such as the liver catabolizes the hormone. The liver may alter the hormone in a number of ways. Its action may result in chemical alterations of the hormone, producing an inactive compound, or the hormone may be so altered that it is more readily excreted from the body. In this way excretion and metabolism of hormones may be interrelated in many instances. Some hormones are readily excreted into the urine, whereas others are excreted into the gastrointestinal tract and into the feces. Some hormones are reabsorbed in the intestines. An enterohepatic circulation of the hormone results when it is secreted in the bile, reabsorbed in the intestinal tract, and then recirculated.

CHEMICAL CLASSIFICATION OF HORMONES

The chemical structure of hormones has been widely investigated over the past 50 years and has been identified for most hormones. For a few of the complex hormonal molecules, however, a detailed chemical structure has not yet been determined. A basic knowledge of chemical structure will help the clinician to select the appropriate assay procedure for determining levels of specific hormones in the circulation. For example, if he is interested in quantitating a growth hormone, the merits of using an immunoassay become obvious.

Basically there are four major chemical classifications of hormones: (1) peptides/polypeptides; (2) amino acid derivatives, i.e., slight modifications of a specific amino acid; (3) steroids; and (4) derivatives of fatty acids. The chemical structure of a hormone determines whether it can be administered orally. If a hormone is a peptide of a relatively large molecular size, it cannot be administered orally, since the normal digestive process would destroy it. However, when one administers the smaller molecular hormone, thyroxine, which is only a slight modification of an amino acid, it is more readily absorbed through the intestinal tract.

ASSAY OF HORMONES

The assay procedures used to determine the level of a specific hormone vary in specificity and sensitivity. The oldest method, the *bioassay*, depends on a biologic response. In this type of assay the hormone is administered to a living system, such as a rat, mouse, or tissue culture. To evaluate the level of the hormone present, a specific response is measured, e.g., cornification of the vaginal mucosa produced by the action of estrogens. However, a bioassay only confirms a hormone's biologic activity; it does not reveal any information about its chemistry. If a clinician is interested in knowing whether the substance has estrogenic activity, a bioassay would be useful. However, if the level of a specific estrogen is to be evaluated, a more sophisticated and detailed assay procedure would be necessary.

In recent years *radioimmunoassay* procedures have come into common usage. These techniques are based on the fact that either the hormone itself can stimulate antibody production when injected into a foreign species, or the hormone is conjugated with material so that the complex (hormone-conjugate) results in antibody formation. Quantitation of the hormone utilizes the specific antibody-antigen reaction. With the addition of tracer amounts of radioactively labeled hormone, these techniques can measure extremely low levels of the material being assayed.

Competitive protein binding assays are techniques that quantitate a substance based on its ability to bind with certain specific proteins. In these procedures a radioactively labeled hormone-plasma protein complex is added. When the hormone to be assayed is added to this mixture, this unlabeled hormone displaces a proportional amount of the radioactive hormone from the complexed material. Quantitation of the released radioactive material permits measurement of the amount of unlabeled hormone that was present originally.

Finally, an assay may involve separation and a specific chemical reaction. These techniques are quite accurate, but they involve long procedures. This type of procedure may incorporate double isotope dilution techniques and/or other procedures in which the material is separated by two or more chromatographic methods. The purified material is then subjected to a specific chemical reaction that permits measurement of the material isolated. Unique physical or chemical properties, such as the absorption of either ultraviolet or visible light, of either the purified hormone itself or the hormone after a chemical reaction, are used as the final quantitation. Gas chromatography can also be used to measure the specific amount of a material after it has been isolated. Addition of a trace amount of radioactive hormone permits correction for losses of the hormone that result from extensive purification during the assay procedure itself.

The clinician should not be too dependent upon a particular assay procedure. The weakness of each type of procedure should be recognized. If an immunoassay procedure is being used, it is important to know whether other hormones, with structures similar to that of the hormone in question, may cross react and thus give a false reading. In the older literature, many investigators reported hormone levels obtained through nonspecific assay procedures. When more precise techniques became available, many of these older writings were found to contain incorrect information. In clinical medicine, because the choice of treatment is based on the results of these studies, it is necessary to make use of the most specific assay procedures possible.

HORMONE EVOLUTION

Through evolution the chemical structure of hormones has changed in many ways from one animal species to another. One way in which a hormone may have evolved is through a change in the way that the hormone is utilized within a specific animal species. For example, prolactin is concerned with lactation in mammals, but may act as a growth hormone in amphibians and reptiles; in certain teleost fish, prolactin appears to be involved in salt and water balance.

Other evolutionary alterations of hormones have resulted in differences in the molecular structure of the hormone in different species. There is a tendency for the mutated or higher form of the hormone to be biologically effective in lower species. However, the original form from lower animals often is inactive in "higher" species. These chemical changes result in species specificity. Human growth hormone has biologic activity in both man and lower animals, but growth hormone from lower animals is not active in man. Changes in the chemical structure of hormones are more readily seen with hormones of the larger molecular size, such as the peptides. However, not all chemical changes alter biologic activity. Although the insulin molecule is somewhat different in structure in many species, such differences do not significantly affect the biologic activity.

PERMISSIVE ACTIONS OF HORMONES

Most hormonal actions are related directly to the amount of hormone present within a certain physiologic range. However, in some instances it appears that a small amount of hormone must be present for a particular body process to function, but the hormone itself does not stimulate the process, and addition of more hormone does not make the process more efficient. This quality has been referred to as the permissive action of hormones. For example, cortisol is necessary for the full action of thyroxine, and insulin is necessary for any actions of growth hormone (GH). However, the permissive action of insulin on GH is not dependent upon GH stimulation of insulin secretion.

PHYSIOLOGIC AND PHARMACOLOGIC LEVELS OF HORMONES

The adage, "if a little is good, a lot must be better," is untrue and dangerous with hormone administration. Physiologic levels of a hormone produce certain well-defined reactions. Nevertheless, if an excessive amount of a hormone is given, very different results may occur. An example of this type of phenomenon is seen with thyroxine, which must be present in physiologic amounts in order for the body to produce protein. Thyroxine, therefore, is protein anabolic. When levels of thyroxine exceed physiologic levels, pharmacologically it becomes protein catabolic and results in the breakdown of protein in the body. Similarly, most hormones, even though necessary for specific reactions in the body, may produce detrimental abnormalities if administered in excessive levels.

PHYSIOLOGIC AND PATHOLOGIC LEVELS OF HORMONES

Pathologic levels of hormones, whether abnormally low or excessively high, are the result of a disease process within the affected animal. If the hormonal levels are high, clinical signs mimic those signs seen when large amounts of the hormone are administered exogenously. The abnormality that results in the pathologic production of a hormone can originate from a specific endocrine tissue. However, pathologic levels of hormones are also produced by nonendocrine tissue, such as certain tumors.

CONTROL OF SECRETION OF HORMONES

In general, increasing secretion of a hormone somewhat reduces further secretion of that particular hormone through a negative feedback mechanism. In addition, as levels of a hormone decrease, release of this feedback mechanism occurs and thus raises the hormonal level to the physiologic range. An example of this negative feedback control mechanism occurs during ACTH stimulation of cortisol secretion. With increasing levels of cortisol in circulation, this steroid inhibits the biosynthesis and release of ACTH. This feedback mechanism for ACTH secretion is mediated through the hypothalamus, where cortisol directly affects the secretion of corticotropin-releasing factor (CRF) from the hypothalamus. CRF is carried through the hypothalamic-pituitary portal venous system to the anterior pituitary gland where it increases the amount of ACTH released. Similarly, thyrotropin (TSH) stimulates thyroxine secretion, but it is the increasing level of thyroxine that results in decreased secretion of TSH. This mechanism is mediated also through the hypothalamus. Through this negative feedback mechanism, the hormones in circulation are maintained within well-defined physiologic levels.

HORMONES SECRETED BY NONENDOCRINE TISSUES

During the last 15 years studies have established that tumors of nonendocrine tissue may secrete hormones or hormone-like materials. If the neoplasm secretes a material that is chemically dissimilar to a specific hormone, but has its exact biologic action, the material is usually referred to as hormone-like material. However, in many instances the material has been discovered to be identical chemically, as well as biologically, to a specific hormone. Researchers have identified a large number of human tumors of nonendocrine tissue that secrete hormone-like materials or hormones themselves. In the dog the most widely identified tumors with this type of capacity have been lymphosarcomas. Lymphosarcomas involving the anterior mediastinum and/or thymus have been shown to secrete a parathormone-like material. I have also seen one case in which lymphosarcoma in a dog resulted in the secretion of ACTH-like material, and thus produced a secondary hyperadrenocorticalism (Cushing's syndrome).

In man — where these abnormalities have been studied in more detail — most of the known hormones have been identified as being secreted by neoplastic tissue of nonendocrine sources. Some of these case reports have been quite unusual; for example, one discusses the secretion of gonadotropins by a hepatoblastoma. This phenomenon is important in certain differential diagnoses. For example, the clinician diagnosing and treating Cushing's syndrome in man must recognize that ACTH is secreted by bronchogenic carcinoma. I believe that further abnormal secretions from tumors will be identified in the dog as more veterinarians realize that these abnormalities exist.

SELECTED READING

1. Aschoff, J.: Comparative physiology: diurnal rhythms. Annu. Rev. Physiol., *25*:581, 1963.
2. Behrle, F. C., Mantz, F. A., Olson, R. L., and Trombold, J. C.: Virilization accompanying hepatoblastoma. Pediatrics, *32*:265, 1963.
3. Boruchow, I. B.: Endocrine and metabolic aspects of bronchogenic carcinoma. Arch. Surg., *90*:101, 1965.
4. Bowers, C. Y.: Studies on the role of cyclic AMP in the release of anterior pituitary hormones. Ann. N.Y. Acad. Sci., *185*:263, 1971.
5. Franchimont, F., Burger, H., and Legros, J. J.: Impact of radioassay techniques on the field of sex hormones. Metabolism, *22*:1003, 1973.
6. Hartiala, K.: Metabolism of hormones, drugs and other substances by the gut. Physiol. Rev., *53*:496, 1973.
7. Hobson, B. M.: The excretion of chorionic gonadotrophin by men with testicular tumors. Acta Endocrinol., *49*:337, 1965.
8. Horai, T., et al.: Oat-cell carcinoma of the lung simultaneously producing ACTH and serotonin. J. Clin. Endocrinol. Metab., *37*:212, 1973.
9. McCann, S. M., Dhariwal, P. S., and Porter, J. C.: Regulation of the adenohypophysis. Annu. Rev. Physiol., *30*:589, 1968.
10. Pang, C. N., and Johnson, D. C.: A method for the preparation of steroid-protein antigens for use in immunoassay of steroids. Steroids, *23*:203, 1974.
11. Pimstone, B. L., Uys, C. J., and Vogelpoel, L.: Studies in a case of Cushing's syndrome due to an ACTH producing thymic tumour. Am. J. Med., *53*:521, 1972.
12. Roth, J.: Peptide hormone binding to receptors: a review of direct studies in vitro. Metabolism, *22*:1059, 1973.
13. Scholz, D. A., et al.: Ectopic hyperparathyroidism with renal calculi and subperiosteal bone resorption. Mayo Clin. Proc., *48*:124, 1973.
14. Skelley, D. S., Brown, L. P., and Besch, P. K.: Radioimmunoassay. Clin. Chem., *19*:146, 1973.

Chapter 2

The Hypothalamus

In addition to being anatomically close to the pituitary, the hypothalamus plays an integrated and important role in controlling the secretions of the adenohypophysis. Much information on hypothalamic control of pituitary secretions has come to light in recent years, and it is now well established that the hypothalamus and the pituitary gland function together as "the master gland." Functions heretofore thought to involve the pituitary alone are now more accurately described as hypothalamic/pituitary functions.

ANATOMY

The hypothalamus has an irregular shape with poorly defined borders (Fig. 2–1). Its anterior portion lies above the optic chiasma and below the anterior commissure; its upper surface extends along the hypothalamic sulcus, which marks the junction of the hypothalamus with the thalamus; its posterior surface, which separates it from the dorsal thalamus, extends from the mamillary bodies below to the foramen of Monro above; and its lateral boundaries, from the top downward, are the internal capsule, the subthalamic nuclei, and the basis pedunculi cerebri.

The hypothalamic nuclei are collections of neurons within the hypothalamus; and in certain areas, some of these neural cells are capable of secreting materials that control the biosynthesis and release of anterior pituitary hormones. Most of these substances have been identified as small peptides, many of which are *releasing factors;* that is, they stimulate the release of anterior pituitary hormonal secretions. Others are *inhibiting factors,* and accordingly inhibit the biosynthesis or release of anterior pituitary hormones.

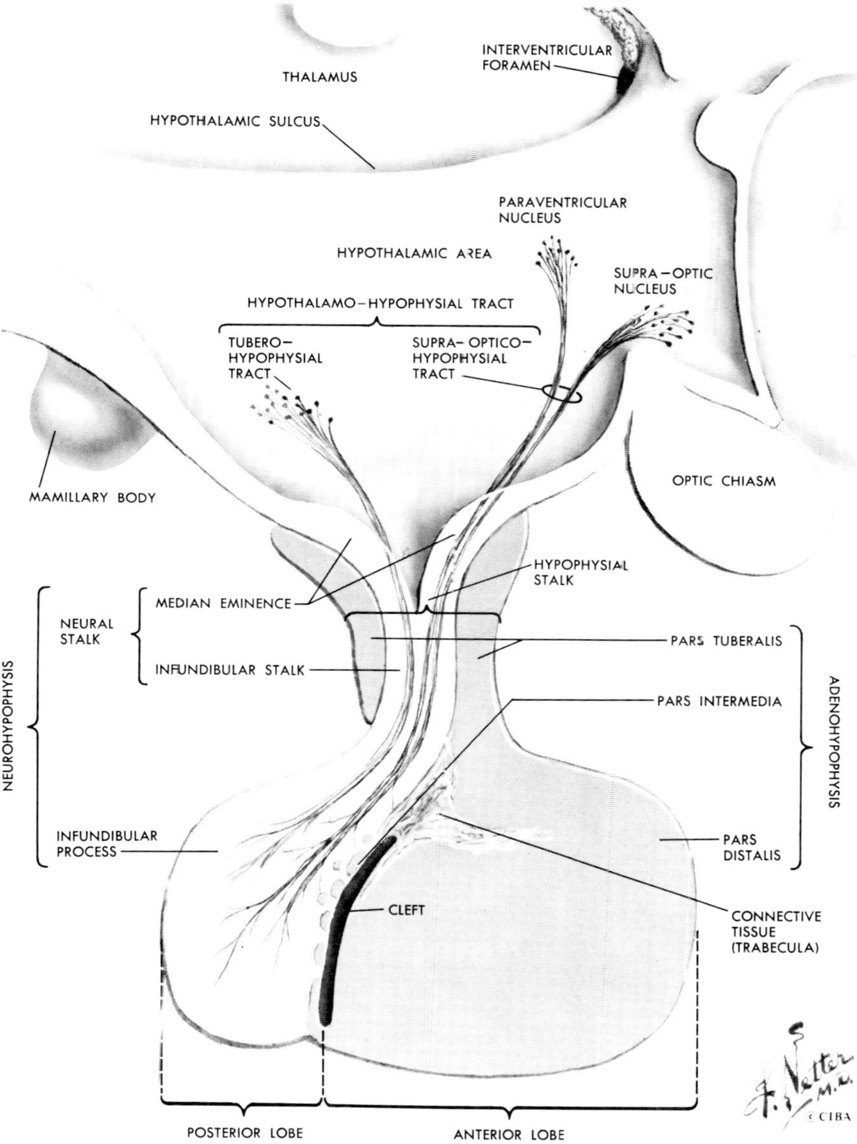

Fig. 2-1. Schematic representation of the hypothalamus and pituitary anatomic relationships. (© Copyright 1955 CIBA Pharmaceutical Company, Division of CIBA-GEIGY Corporation. Reproduced with permission from THE CIBA COLLECTION OF MEDICAL ILLUSTRATIONS by Frank H. Netter, M.D. All rights reserved.)

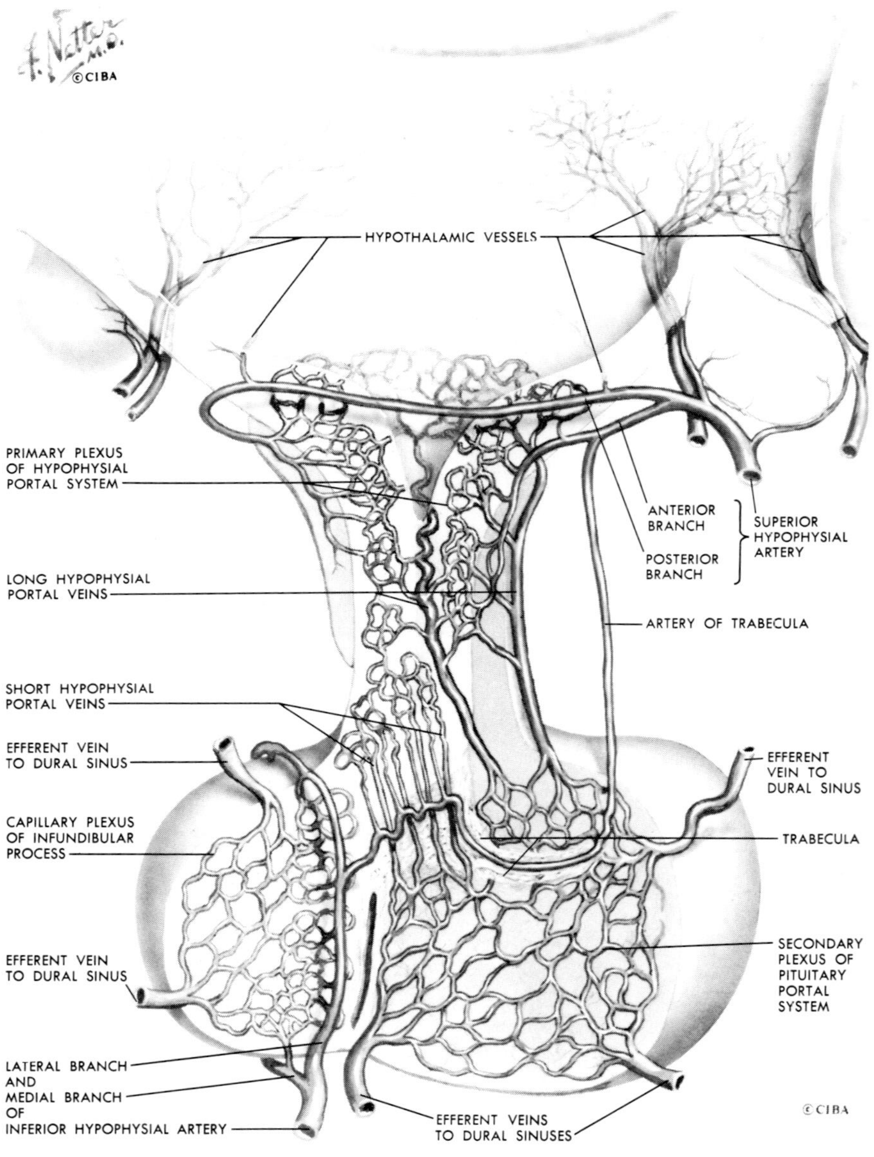

Fig. 2–2. Schematic representation of the blood supply to the hypothalamus and pituitary gland. (© Copyright 1965 CIBA Pharmaceutical Company, Division of CIBA-GEIGY Corporation. Reproduced with permission from THE CIBA COLLECTION OF MEDICAL ILLUSTRATIONS by Frank H. Netter, M.D. All rights reserved.)

Other specific nuclei in the hypothalamus control posterior pituitary function, but by a different mechanism from that described for control of the anterior pituitary. Posterior pituitary function originates with the synthesis of *vasopressin* (ADH) and *oxytocin*, respectively, inside the supraoptic and paraventricular nuclei within the hypothalamus. These hormones, along with a carrier protein substance, are transmitted down axons to the posterior pituitary, where they are released at the nerve endings to be further distributed to their target organs.

The effect of the hypothalamic neurosecretions on the anterior pituitary gland is not under direct nervous system control, as is the case with the posterior pituitary. Instead the neurosecretions are carried by an elaborate and specialized venous portal system (composed of vascular connections) between the hypothalamus and the anterior pituitary (Fig. 2–2). The anterior pituitary receives little direct arterial blood supply. Most of the blood reaching it is carried first by arterioles to the hypothalamus. Within the hypothalamus the vessels branch into a network of capillaries, which transport the neurohumoral secretions from the hypothalamus. The capillaries and venules coalesce into slightly larger vessels to make up the portal plexus, which carries the blood directly to the anterior pituitary. In the adenohypophysis the portal vessels again divide into capillaries, which carry the releasing and inhibiting factors.

PHYSIOLOGY

In addition to its important function as regulator of the anterior pituitary gland, the hypothalamus regulates other important functions such as body temperature, sleep, and appetite. An increasing number of releasing and inhibiting factors has been isolated and identified from the hypothalamus in recent years. Since many of these substances have a relatively simple chemical structure, they have been synthesized and are becoming available for experimental and chemical research. Although they have not yet gained a place in the everyday picture of veterinary medicine, it appears that this will soon be the case. Since the availability of these factors is limited at present, they are being used mainly by the research endocrinologist in human medicine. The use of these substances for diagnostic purposes is expected to help in defining specific abnormalities in the hypothalamus, in the pituitary, and in the target tissue itself.

Substances now undergoing active investigation include *corticotropin-releasing factor* (CRF), which stimulates the release of adrenocorticotropin (ACTH); *thyrotropin-releasing factor* (TRF), which controls the secretion of thyrotropin (TSH); *prolactin-inhibiting factor* (PIF), which is involved in the secretion of prolactin; and *somatostatin* or somatotropin-inhibiting factor (SIF).

Releasing and inhibiting factors for the gonadotropins have been identified in a number of species. As the evidence accumulates, it appears likely that a releasing factor and/or an inhibiting factor exist to control secretion of most, if not all, of the anterior pituitary hormones.

ABNORMALITIES

Hypofunction or hyperfunction of the anterior pituitary gland may originate with disease within the gland itself or with abnormal function of the hypothalamus. For example, an insufficiency of thyrotropin (pituitary hypothyroidism) may be the result of either an insufficiency of thyrotropin itself within the pituitary, or an insufficiency of thyrotropin-releasing factor from the hypothalamus. It is not always possible to differentiate between the two types of disorders clinically, but such differentiation may become commonplace when commercially prepared releasing and inhibiting factors are readily applied to clinical medicine.

Hypogonadism resulting from an insufficiency of gonadotropin secretion could also result from either a direct pituitary insufficiency or hypothalamic disease. It is reasonable to expect that all abnormalities once considered to be pituitary in origin could result from an insufficiency of specific releasing factors, an excessive secretion of releasing factors, an increased secretion of inhibiting factors, or an insufficiency of inhibiting factors.

An insufficient state of the posterior pituitary gland can be the result of a lesion or abnormality of the supraoptic nuclei in the hypothalamus. The lesion may cause an insufficiency of ADH and, consequently, diabetes insipidus, which is characterized by an extreme increase in water diuresis. The dog so afflicted excretes liters of urine with low specific gravity, usually below 1.004. The normal physiologic stimuli to the secretion of ADH, such as water deprivation, fail to produce an increased secretion of ADH. Therefore, the kidney is unable to reabsorb the water that normally would be controlled by the action of ADH in the kidney tubules and collecting ducts. Diabetes insipidus can result from a destructive lesion in the hypothalamus itself — a lesion that would interrupt the axons which traverse the pituitary stalk, or one that would destroy the posterior pituitary lobe. This disorder will be described in more detail in Chapter 6.

Just as pituitary and/or hypothalamic disorders are occasionally difficult to separate from one another, it is equally difficult to pinpoint the cause in some cases of *obesity*. Two distinct mechanisms in the hypothalamus can be held accountable. If the area affected controls the release of TRF, an insufficiency of this factor causes a decrease in the secretion of thyrotropin, which in turn decreases the secretion of thyroid hormone. This type of secondary hypothyroidism produces a decreased metabolic rate, and the animal so affected usually has a normal or slightly less than normal appetite. The other form of hypothalamic obesity can be caused by a destructive lesion in the area that controls appetite. In this case the obese animal has a voracious appetite. The latter type of obesity is rare in the dog, although in most cases the obesity does result from the intake of excessive amounts of food. In the few documented cases of excessive appetite due to hypothalamic disease, a sudden change in the amount of food intake has been noted. Rarely would this type of polyphagia be present throughout the lifetime of these dogs.

Lactational abnormalities are common in the dog. Occasionally spaying a bitch during diestrus results in the sudden development of lactorrhea. Although the specific mechanism for this excessive lactation is not known, it is possible that hypothalamic and/or anterior pituitary gland dysfunction may be the cause. One explanation is that excessive secretion of prolactin occurs following spaying at a critical time during the estrous cycle. This type of lactational abnormality, although bothersome, may take eight to ten weeks to regress. It usually does not in itself cause problems other than discomfort for the bitch.

SELECTED READING

1. Bogdanove, E. M.: Regulation of thyroidal function. Fed. Proc., *21*:623, 1962.
2. Endroczi, E., and Hilliard, J.: Luteinizing hormone releasing activity in different parts of rabbit and dog brain. Endocrinology, *77*:667, 1965.
3. Everett, J. W.: Central neural control of reproductive functions of the adenohypophysis. Physiol. Rev., *44*:373, 1964.
4. Greep, R. O.: A vista of research on the mammalian gonadotropins. Biol. Reprod., *8*:2, 1973.
5. Greep, R. O.: The gonadotrophins and their releasing factors. J. Reprod. Fertil. [Suppl.], *20*:1, 1973.
6. Guillemin, R.: Hypothalamic polypeptides releasing pituitary hormones. Metabolism, *13*:1206, 1964.
7. Guillemin, R.: The adenohypophysis and its hypothalamic control. Annu. Rev. Physiol., *29*:313, 1967.
8. McCann, S. M., Ramirez, V. D., and Igarashi, M.: Hypothalamic FSH and LH-releasing factors. Metabolism, *13*:1177, 1964.
9. Meites, J., and Nicoll, C. S.: Adenohypophysis: prolactin. Annu. Rev. Physiol., *28*:57, 1966.
10. Netter, F. H.: The Ciba Collection of Medical Illustrations. Endocrine System and Selected Metabolic Diseases. Ciba Pharmaceutical Company, *4*:4, 1965.
11. Paschkis, K. E., Rakoff, A. E., Cantarow, A., and Rupp, J. J.: Clinical Endocrinology. 3rd ed. Harper & Row, New York, 1967, p. 13.
12. Schally, A. V., et al.: Chromatography and hormonal activities of dog hypothalamus. Endocrinology, *70*:478, 1962.
13. Sloper, J. C., and Bateson, R.: Ultrastructure of neurosecretory cells in the supraoptic nucleus of the dog and rat. J. Endocrinol., *31*:139, 1965.
14. Wurster, D. H., and Benirschke, K.: Development of the hypothalamo-hypophysial neurosecretory system in the fetal armadillo (Dasypus novemcinctus) with notes on rabbit, cat and dog. Gen. Comp. Endocrinol., *4*:433, 1964.
15. Zarrow, M. X., Gandelman, R., and Dennenberg, V. H. Prolactin: is it an essential hormone for maternal behavior in the mammal? Horm. Behav., *2*:343, 1971.

Chapter

3

The Anterior Pituitary Gland

ANATOMY

The pituitary gland originates embryonically from two ectodermal sources. One is a ventral outgrowth from the floor of the diencephalon; the other an upward growth of Rathke's pouch from the roof of the oral cavity. The two join to form the neurohypophysis (posterior pituitary lobe) and the adenohypophysis (the anterior lobe) respectively. As differentiation proceeds, both derivatives become subdivided into several specialized zones, more or less distinct structurally and functionally. The vascular supply to the anterior pituitary gland is mainly through the portal venous network, which carries blood from the hypothalamic area. This portal system transmits neurohumoral factors to the anterior pituitary gland. These releasing and inhibiting factors, which are produced in the hypothalamus, control the ultimate function of the anterior pituitary gland.

HISTOLOGY

The histologic composition of the anterior pituitary has been described in detail in recent years. From a functional standpoint it can be somewhat simplified. Basically there are two major types of cells, differentiated by their affinity for specific dyes. The staining properties of the cells are best demonstrated by procedures using eosin and methyl blue. The cells that do not readily stain are called chromophobe cells. These cells are fairly abundant, and are believed to be the cells that secrete adrenocorticotropin (ACTH). The cells that do stain well are the chromophil cells. The red-staining cells are the acidophils, and the blue-staining cells the basophils. The use of hematoxylin and eosin staining often gives poor differentiation of the acidophils and basophils. The acidophils are believed to secrete growth hormone (GH) and prolactin (LTH). The basophils are the cells considered to secrete thyrotropin (TSH), gonadotropins (FSH and LH), and possibly melanocyte-stimulating hormone (MSH).

Although this classification based on histologic appearance may be somewhat simplified, it does assist in correlating certain tumors and degenerative lesions of the anterior pituitary with specific disorders. Acidophilic adenomas and adenocarcinomas, both GH-secreting tumors, are rare in the dog. The basophilic adenoma and adenocarcinoma have been described more frequently. In the older literature the basophilic tumors were thought to be the cause of Cushing's disease in man and dog. With sensitive assay procedures for ACTH now available, it has been shown that it is the chromophobic tumor that secretes ACTH. Plasma levels of ACTH have been found to be low when basophilic tumors are present with hyperadrenocorticalism. It is thought by some investigators that basophilic tumors, when present with Cushing's syndrome, may be the result of the high levels of corticosteroid secretion, rather than the cause of it.

PHYSIOLOGY

Any discussion of the anterior pituitary lobe in the dog must be qualified by the fact that most information cited has not been obtained from studies in the dog itself. Pituitary function has been mainly studied in man or laboratory animals, such as the rat or mouse.

The gonadotropins—follicle-stimulating hormone (FSH), luteinizing hormone (LH) or interstitial cell-stimulating hormone (ICSH)—and thyrotropin (TSH) are glycoproteins. In recent years one question has been whether the gonadotropins were secreted as two separate hormones or were the result of metabolism of one larger molecule. It has been demonstrated, at least to my satisfaction, that the mammalian anterior pituitary gland secretes FSH and LH as two different molecular entities. Both gonadotropins have been prepared chemically; and their amino acid and carbohydrate composition is known in some species. Recent studies have demonstrated that the gonadotropins may be separated into two subunits — now referred to as the alpha and beta subunits. Of the glycoprotein hormones that have been studied in detail to date, the alpha subunits are remarkably similar. The sequence of the complete molecule of FSH has not been settled, but it appears from present evidence that the alpha subunit of FSH differs slightly from the alpha subunit of LH. These subunits have little biologic activity themselves, usually only 1 or 2% of the activity of the native molecule. However, when the subunits are combined, complete activity is restored. Since the alpha subunits are nearly identical, the nature of the activity is actually determined by the beta subunit.

An abundance of evidence suggests that one factor is responsible for the release of both LH and FSH. However, this fact still remains somewhat controversial. The response to other releasing factors is hormone-specific in that thyrotropin-releasing hormone (TRH) and corticotropin-releasing hormone (CRF) do not release gonadotropins, and conversely. Essentially, the evidence seems to be that the releasing factors are not species-specific. In addition, releasing factors stimulate synthesis as well as the release of the hormones.

The hypothalamic neurohumoral substance that increases the secretion rate of ACTH is CRF. The CRF from stalk-median eminence tissue is probably the material that has most physiologic significance. Cortisol, the major adrenal glucocorticoid in the dog, is the main factor in the negative feedback mechanism. When the level of cortisol increases in the circulation, it has an inhibiting effect on the release of CRF. This reaction produces a decreased secretion of ACTH, and restoration of the plasma cortisol to its lower physiologic level.

Thyrotropin-releasing facator (TRF) is under active investigation. Its chemical structure is known; and being a small peptide, it has become available for clinical and basic research. In the dog, free thyroxine in the plasma appears to be the important hormone in the negative feedback mechanism. It has not been established whether triiodothyronine is a physiologic hormone in the dog[1] although this potent hormone in man[2,3,4] has been isolated in dog blood.[5] However, studies demonstrating that it has biologic activity in the canine are not convincing. It appears that T_3 probably has little effect, if any, on the feedback mechanism and the release of thyrotropin.

Simply stated, FSH stimulates ovarian follicle growth and maturation in the female. In the male, FSH, along with testosterone, is necessary for spermatogenesis. LH in the female stimulates the formation of the corpus luteum, and with FSH, it stimulates estrogen secretion. It is also necessary for ovulation. Some of the actions of the gonadotropins vary from species to species. In the dog, the requisite presence of FSH, LH, or both for estrogen secretion has not been well studied. In some species LH is necessary for the complete effect of FSH on follicular development. In the male, LH is also called interstitial cell-stimulating hormone (ICSH). ICSH stimulates the interstitial cells of the testes to produce testosterone, and FSH may enhance this function.

Prolactin (luteotropic hormone or LTH) maintains lactation in the female; and in some species it also stimulates the corpus luteum to secrete progesterone. In some species, prolactin is called luteotropin (LTH) because it stimulates progesterone secretion by the corpus luteum, whereas in other species prolactin has little effect on the maintenance of progesterone secretion. To my knowledge, the action of prolactin on progesterone secretion in the dog is not known. Prolactin action in the male appears to have a direct stimulatory effect on prostatic growth. This action is probably synergistic with the action of testosterone on prostatic tissue.

TSH stimulates the biosynthesis of thyroid hormones. It also stimulates the growth of the thyroid by increasing cell size and cell number. TSH stimulates the increased uptake of iodine by the thyroid, and increases its incorporation into thyroglobulin within the thyroid follicle. The hydrolysis of thyroglobulin and the release of thyroxine into the circulation are also enhanced by TSH.

ACTH stimulates the adrenal cortex to secrete mainly cortisol, other corticosteroids, and some androgens as well. ACTH is necessary for the maintenance of normal adrenal size. In man, ACTH will increase pigmentation because part of the molecule of ACTH is similar to the alpha-MSH (Fig. 3–1). However, ACTH does not cause pigmentation in the dog. Even when ACTH levels are high, pigmentation does not occur in the dog. For example, following adrenalectomy, if glucocorticoid replacement is absent, plasma ACTH levels in the blood increase, but pigmentation does not occur.

Growth hormone (somatotropin or GH) produces general tissue growth without maturation. Each species seems to have a different molecular composition of its GH, and the response to a given GH preparation varies. GH stimulates growth of the long bones provided the epiphyses are open. Protein anabolism mediated through suppression of amino-acid catabolism is an important GH function. GH also facilitates transport of amino acids into cells. The "anti-insulin effect" of GH is believed to be mediated through an interference with phosphorylation of glucose; therefore, it is considered to be

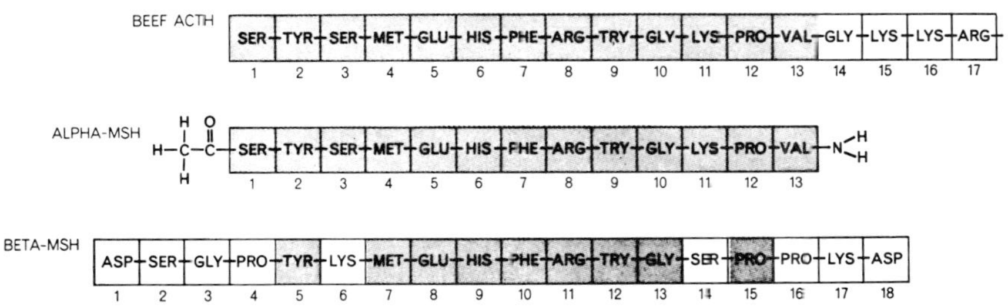

Fig. 3–1. Partial schematic formula of beef ACTH; 1 through 17 subunits (top) of the total 39 subunit ACTH structure is shown. Except for two small chemical details, alpha-MSH is identical with the first 13 subunits in natural ACTH. Of the 18 subunits in beta-MSH, half coincide with those in the first 12 subunits of ACTH. (From "The ACTH Molecule" by Choh Hao Li: Copyright © 1963 by Scientific American, Inc. All rights reserved.)

diabetogenic. Bovine GH has biologic activity in the dog, and excessive administration of exogenous GH has been shown experimentally to produce a permanent diabetes mellitus in the dog after only a few weeks (Fig. 3–2). This disease was experimentally produced using bovine GH. However, if the bovine GH was administered for less than two weeks, the diabetes was transient. The blood glucose returned to normal when the administration of GH was terminated (Fig. 3–3). Whether excessive administration of canine GH would produce permanent diabetes mellitus as readily as bovine GH remains to be seen. This diabetogenic effect of GH can be demonstrated only in the adult dog. Puppies do not become diabetic when exogenous GH is administered.

An interesting comparison was formulated years ago when discussing diabetes mellitus that occurred in people secondary to an excessive secretion of GH. Physicians often designated whether the person with this type of diabetes mellitus was "dog-like" or "rat-like." Diabetes mellitus produced in the dog following the administration of excessive GH is usually permanent, and even though GH is no longer being administered, the dog continues to be diabetic. The disease is

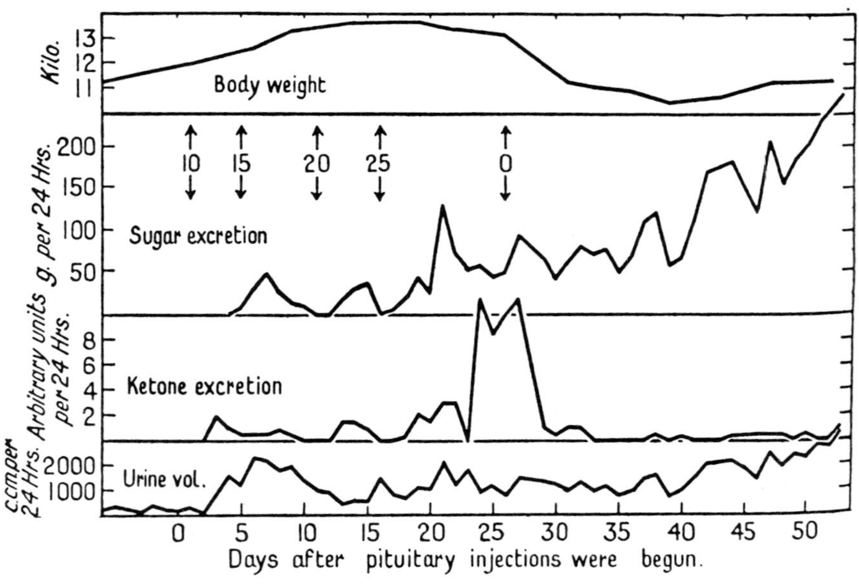

Fig. 3–2. Permanent diabetes produced by pituitary extract in the dog. The figures on the arrows give the weight of fresh ox anterior lobe used to prepare the amount of extract injected daily, from the day indicated by the arrow, onward. Injections were stopped on day 26. (From Young, F. G.: Lancet, 2:372, 1937.)

Effect of anterior pituitary extract on the insulin content of pancreas and average blood-sugar level.

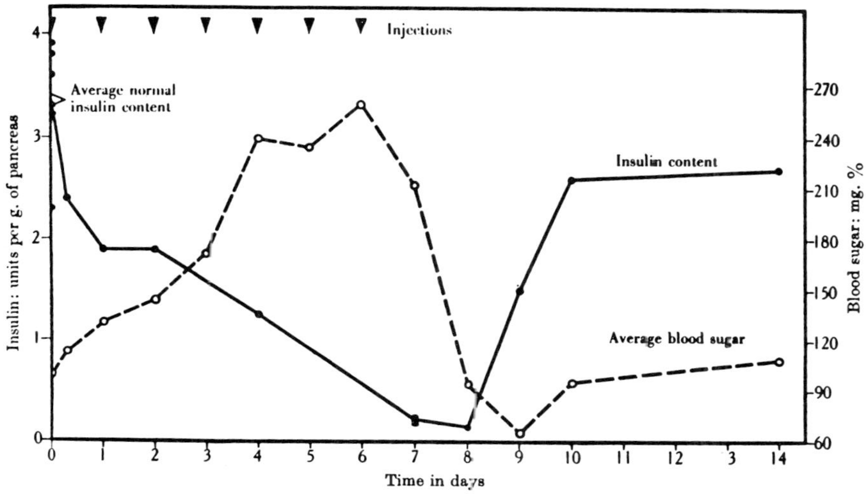

Fig. 3–3. Reversible diabetes produced by anterior pituitary extract in the dog. Blood sugar and insulin content of pancreas. (From Best, C. H., Campbell, J., and Haist, R. E.: J. Physiol., 97:203, 1939, Cambridge University Press.)

irreversible. In rats, however, diabetes mellitus produced by the administration of excessive GH abates when GH administration is discontinued. The rat is more readily able to revert to a normal state. Therefore, if persons with pituitary gigantism and/or acromegaly (excessive GH secretion) develop diabetes mellitus, and if the diabetes disappears following correction of the excessive GH secretion, they are considered rat-like. If diabetes does not correct itself and is permanent, these individuals are considered dog-like.

PATHOLOGY

The most commonly reported abnormality of the canine pituitary gland is the neoplasm. However, in my experience, many functional disorders of the pituitary are not associated with neoplasms. In fact, altered functional pituitary disorders can occur without any gross or histologic abnormality.

The most common pituitary tumor reported in the dog is the chromophobic adenoma or adenocarcinoma. Less frequently observed is the basophilic adenoma or adenocarcinoma. The acidophilic tumor is rarely reported. Other degenerative pituitary lesions have been reported occasionally, but abnormalities such as postpartum pituitary necrosis, similar to the Simmonds and Sheehan syndromes in man, have not been reported in the dog. This latter disorder usually is associated with general circulatory collapse and postpartum hemorrhage. In women with this disorder, thrombosis and necrosis of the anterior pituitary gland occur and result in panhypopituitarism. Clinical signs usually become evident after parturition. Attempts to produce it experimentally in the dog have not been successful.

Other histopathologic abnormalities of the canine pituitary gland have been described. However, it should be emphasized that the important aspect of an endocrine disease is the functional status of that particular endocrine gland. This status need not be associated with any specific pathologic finding. In other words, it is of little consequence whether the tissue appears normal if the functional state is abnormal. Although the pituitary gland may appear to be normal on histologic examination, an endocrine disorder is nevertheless present if an insufficiency or an excess secretion exists.

EFFECT OF ANTERIOR PITUITARY HORMONE ON OTHER METABOLIC PROCESSES

The interaction of hormones is a complex process. Rarely does a single hormone influence a metabolic process. In fact, interaction of hormones occurs in most metabolic processes within the body. Since some of these factors are important clinically, they will be considered in the discussions of the pathogenesis of the endocrine diseases.

One particularly important interaction, discussed earlier, is the fact that administration of bovine GH in excess to dogs results in the development of diabetes mellitus. If GH is given for less than two weeks, the hyperglycemia is reversible. However, with GH injections for three weeks or more, a permanent diabetes results. It appears that the canine pancreas is unable to recover normally. The hyperglycemia is the result of interference with the GH transport of glucose into cells. This condition stimulates insulin secretion. However, in the dog the pancreas does not continue oversecreting, but instead appears to progress into a state of exhaustion atrophy. When this state occurs, insulin secretion decreases to low levels. Conversely, the pituitary dwarf who has an insufficiency of GH is especially sensitive to the action of insulin. This increased insulin sensitivity may be reversed by administering GH. The influence of the anterior pituitary gland on carbohydrate metabolism, and the mechanism of its diabetogenic action, are the result of a number of interactions. Only growth hormone has been discussed to this point. The effects of the anterior pituitary gland mediated through stimulation of the adrenal cortex and thyroid gland are other aspects that must be considered. In following chapters many of these facets will be discussed in more detail.

REFERENCES

1. Roberts, K. E., et al.: Effect of phosphate in enhancing the action of triiodothyronine. Endocrinology, *59*:565, 1956.
2. Patel, Y. C., and Burger, H. G.: Serum triiodothyronine in health and disease. Clin. Endocrinol., *2*:339, 1973.
3. Singer, P. A., and Nicoloff, J. T.: Estimation of the triiodothyronine secretion rate in euthyroid man. J. Clin. Endocrinol. Metab., *35*:82, 1972.
4. Nagataki, S., et al.: Triiodothyronine and thyroxine in thyroid glands of euthyroid Japanese subjects. J. Clin. Endocrinol. Metab., *35*:18, 1972.
5. Taurog, A., Porter, J. C., and Thio, D. T.: Nature of the ^{131}I-compounds released into the thyroid veins of rabbits, dogs and cats before and after TSH administration. Endocrinology, *74*:902, 1964.

SELECTED READING

1. Altszuler, N., Rathgeb, I., Winkler, B., and deBodo, R. C.: The effects of growth hormone on carbohydrate and lipid metabolism in the dog. Ann. N. Y. Acad. Sci., *148*:441, 1968.
2. Andersen, R. N., and Egdahl, R. H.; Effect of vasopressin on pituitary-adrenal secretion in the dog. Endocrinology, *74*:538, 1964.
3. Best, C. H., Campbell, J., and Haist, R. E.: Effects of anterior pituitary extracts on insulin content of pancreas. J. Physiol., *97*:200, 1939.
4. Bishop, J. S., et al.: Diminished responsiveness to insulin in the growth hormone-treated normal dog. Am. J. Physiol., *212*:272, 1967.
5. Capen, C. C., Martin, S. L., and Koestner, A.: Neoplasms in the adenohypophysis of dogs. A clinical and pathologic study. Pathol. Vet., *4*:301, 1967.
6. Capen, C. C., and Koestner, A.: Functional chromophobe adenomas of the canine adenohypophysis. An ultrastructural evaluation of a neoplasm of the pituitary corticotrophs. Pathol. Vet., *4*:326, 1967.
7. Egdahl, R. H.: The acute effects of steroid administration on pituitary-adrenal secretion in the dog. J. Clin. Invest., *43*:2178, 1964.
8. Francis, K. C., and Mulligan, R. M.: The weight of the pituitary gland of the male dog in relation to body weight and age with a differential cell count of the anterior lobe. J. Morphol., *85*:141, 1949.
9. Gans, J. H., and Butz, R. L.: Comparative effects of growth hormone: cholesterol metabolism and the composition of plasma, liver, and bile in dogs treated with growth hormone. Am. J. Vet. Res., *25*:1695, 1964.
10. Goldberg, R. C., and Chailsoff, I. L.: On the occurrence of six cell types in the dog anterior pituitary. Anat. Rec., *112*:265, 1952.
11. Greep, R. O.: The gonadotrophins and their releasing factors. J. Reprod. Fertil. [Suppl.] *20*:1, 1973.
12. Groen, J. J., Frenkel, H. S., and Offerhous, L.: Observations on a case of spontaneous diabetes mellitus in a dog. Diabetes, *13*:492, 1964.
13. Guillemin, R.: The adenohypophysis and its hypothalamic control. Annu. Rev. Physiol., *29*:313, 1967.
14. Hartree, A. S., Bell, E. T., Christie, D. W., and Kirkham, K. E.: Partial purification of dog pituitary glycoprotein hormones. J. Endocrinol., *52*:403, 1972.
15. Hashimoto, C., et al.: Purification and characterization of growth hormone from dog pituitary glands. Endocrinology, *88*:381, 1971.
16. Hewitt, W. F., Jr.: Age and sex differences in weight of pituitary gland in dogs. Proc. Soc. Exp. Biol. Med., *74*:781, 1950.
17. Hightower, D., Kyzar, J. R., Chester, D. K., and Wright, E. M.: Replacement therapy for induced hypothyroidism in dogs. J. Am. Vet. Med. Assoc., *163*:979, 1973.

18. King, J. M., Kavanaugh, J. F., and Bentinck-Smith, J.: Diabetes mellitus with pituitary neoplasms in a horse and a dog. The Cornell Vet., *52*:133, 1962.
19. Kovach, A. G. B., Monos, E., and Edit, K.: Adrenal blood flow and corticosteroid secretion: II. The effect of oxytocin on adrenal blood flow and corticoid secretion before and after acute hypophysectomy in the dog. Acta Physiol. (Hungary), *28*:155, 1965.
20. Kral, F.: Treatment of some acquired alopecic and acanthotic skin disorders in dogs. Small Anim. Clinician, *3*:427, 1963.
21. Latimer, H. B.: The weight of the hypophysis in the dog. Growth, *5*:293, 1941.
22. Li, C. H.: The ACTH molecule. Sci. Am., *209*:46, 1963.
23. McCann, S. M., Ramirez, V. D., and Igarashi, M.: Hypothalamic FSH and LH-releasing factors. Metabolism, *13*:1189, 1964.
24. Meier, H.: Etiologic considerations of spontaneous tumors in animals with special reference to the endocrine system. Ann. N. Y. Acad. Sci., *108*:881, 1963.
25. Morgan, M., Altszuler, N., and Rathgeb, I.: Failure of injected growth hormone to increase plasma glucose and insulin concentration in the puppy. Endocrinology, *96*:538, 1975.
26. Mulligan, R. M.: Neoplasms of the Dog. Williams & Wilkins, Baltimore, 1949.
27. Rathgeb, I., Winkler, B., Steele, R., and Altszuler, N.: Effects of canine growth hormone on the metabolism of plasma glucose and free fatty acids in the dog. Endocrinology, *87*:628, 1970.
28. Rathgeb, I., Steele, R., Winkler, B., and Altszuler, N.: Influence of fasting on changes in glucose metabolism induced by growth hormone injection in the normal dog. Diabetes, *19*:487, 1970.
29. Rovit, R. L., and Duane, T. D.: Cushing's syndrome and pituitary tumors. Am. J. Med., *46*:416, 1969.
30. Siegel, E. T.: Assessment of pituitary-adrenal gland function in the dog. Am. J. Vet. Res., *29*:173, 1968.
31. Sokolowski, J. H., Medernach, R. W., and Helper, L. C.: Exogenous hormone therapy to control the estrous cycle of the bitch. J. Am. Vet. Med. Assoc., *153*:425, 1968.
32. Tsushima, T., Irie, M., and Sakuma, M.: Radioimmunoassay for canine growth hormone. Endocrinology, *89*:685, 1971.
33. Updike, G. B., Jr., and Corey, E. L.: Experimental attempts to produce anterior pituitary necrosis in the rat and dog. Am. J. Obstet. Gynecol., *90*:25, 1964.
34. Wagle, S. R., and Gans, J. H.: Effects of growth hormone on glucose-U-C^{14} metabolism in dog. Proc. Soc. Exp. Biol. Med., *116*:793, 1964.
35. White, J. B., and Foust, H. L.: Growth changes in body organs. III. Growth changes in the pituitary of the normal dogs. Am. J. Vet. Res., *5*:173, 1944.
36. Wilhelmi, A. E.: Canine growth hormone. Yale J. Biol. Med., *41*:199, 1968.
37. Young, F. G.: Permanent experimental diabetes produced by pituitary (anterior lobe) injections. Lancet, *2*:372, 1937.

Chapter 4

Hypofunction of the Anterior Pituitary Gland

PITUITARY DWARFISM

Pituitary dwarfism is the abnormality resulting from an insufficiency of growth hormone (GH) during the growing phase of an animal. This type of dwarfism is readily distinguishable from other types of dwarfism. With pituitary dwarfism the animal is small in size, but is normal in its proportions (Figs. 4–1 and 4–2). There may be

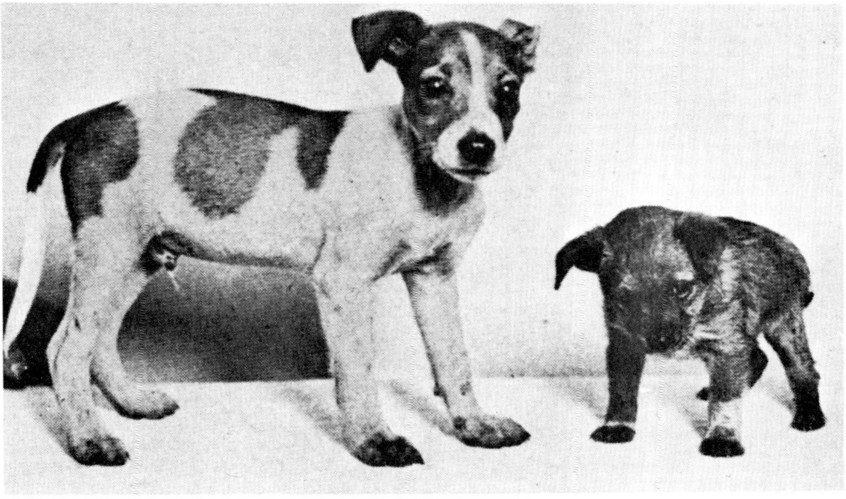

Fig. 4–1. Experimentally produced pituitary dwarf. Hypophysectomized puppy (right) and its littermate control (left). Dogs are four months of age. Hypophysectomy was carried out at three weeks of age. (From Dandy, W. E., and Reichert, F. L.: Bull. Johns Hopkins Hosp., 62:129, 1938.)

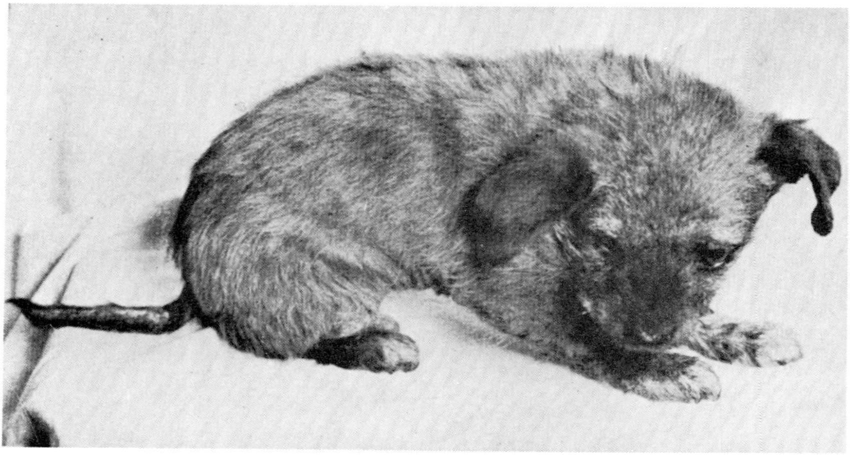

Fig. 4–2. Close-up showing hypophysectomized puppy in Fig. 4–1 at nine months of age. (From Dandy, W. E., and Reichert, F. L.: Bull. Johns Hopkins Hosp., *62*:131, 1938.)

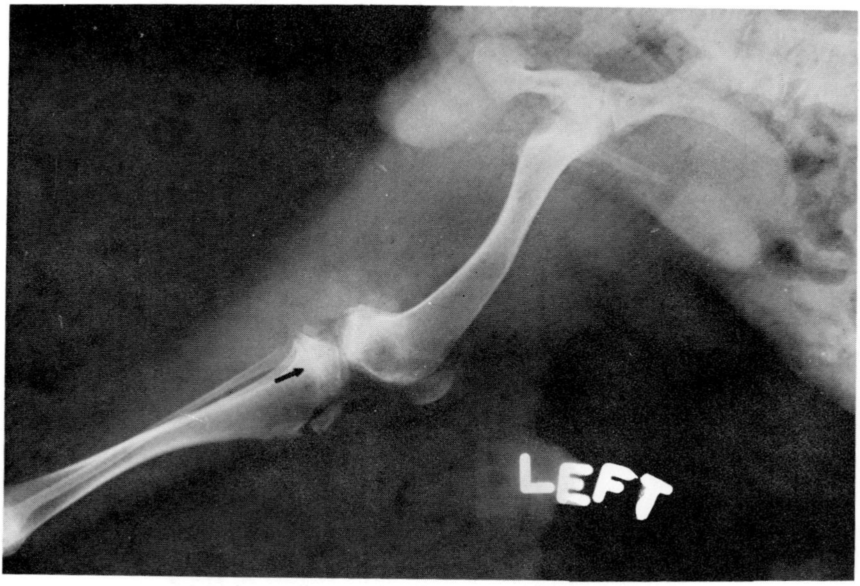

Fig. 4–3. Lateral radiograph of the femur and tibia of a 13-month-old pituitary dwarf. The epiphyseal lines of the long bones remain open, indicating that the bone age is less than the actual age.

almost total cessation of growth of long bones, and the epiphyseal lines do not close normally. There is an appreciable delay in epiphyseal closure. In the normal dog, depending on the breed and the specific long bone, normal closure of most long bones occurs between seven and twelve months of age. In the pituitary dwarf, the epiphyses are usually open well beyond the age of 1½ years (Fig. 4–3). The epiphyses do close even if untreated, but this closure frequently does not occur until three or four years of age. The variation of closure time appears to be dependent upon the severity of the insufficiency of GH.

In man a sensitive and precise immunoassay is available for GH. However, in the dog, since only limited amounts of purified dog GH are available, assay of GH is not routinely carried out. Since the assay procedure is not widely available, the diagnosis of canine pituitary dwarfism is based on the clinical signs and radiographic findings.

Canine pituitary dwarfs remain infantile not only in growth, but also in other functions. They retain their soft puppy-like haircoat and shrill bark. Their first dentition is retained longer than normal, and the genitalia are often infantile (Figs. 4–4 and 4–5). Regrowth of hair following clipping or shaving takes at least twice as long as normal. In

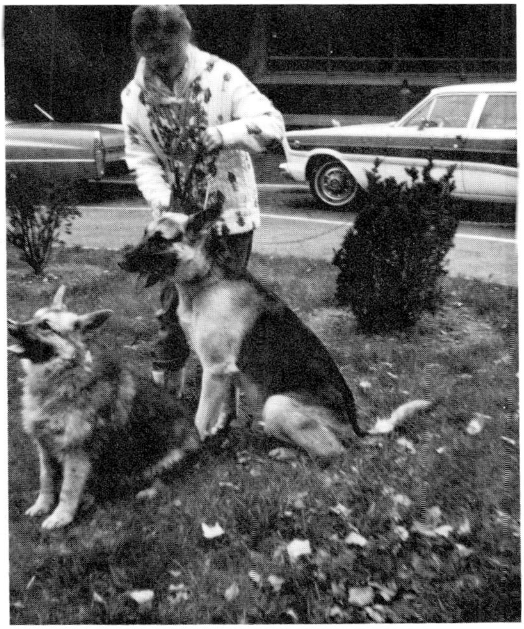

Fig. 4–4. Panhypopituitary German shepherd dwarf 2½ years of age and its normal littermate.

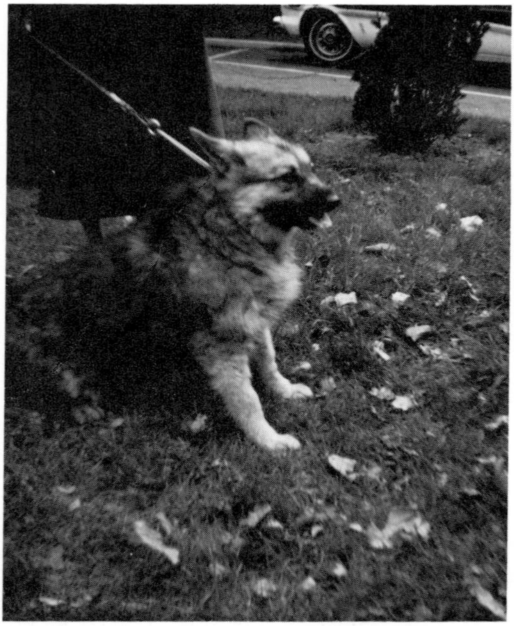

Fig. 4–5. Close-up of panhypopituitary German shepherd dwarf shown in Fig. 4–4. Note the soft puppy-like haircoat and the immature appearance.

the complete absence of GH, regrowth of hair following clipping may not occur at all.

Another clinical sign that might assist in making an earlier clinical diagnosis in the male dog relates to the fact that the os penis is dependent on GH and androgens for normal calcification. In the normal male dog the os penis calcifies at about four to five months of age. Complete calcification of the os penis in the pituitary dwarf is delayed. Clinically, when I examine a canine dwarf of one year of age or more with incomplete calcification of the os penis, I make a tentative diagnosis of pituitary dwarfism.

Treatment of canine pituitary dwarfism depends on the availability of GH. Bovine GH is effective in the dog. However, since bovine GH is not effective in man, it has become almost as difficult to obtain as canine GH. I believe that human GH is effective in the dog, but it has not been proven. Human GH has been synthesized in the laboratory in recent years, and the availability of human GH for clinical use in the future does appear probable. It should be noted, however, that most owners of canine pituitary dwarfs do not dislike the general appearance or size of the animal. Most owners actually prefer the miniature size. They usually seek veterinary attention when hair begins to fall out.

Although regrowth of the haircoat after clipping is seen early in the course of the disease, the dog will begin to lose hair even if the hair is not cut. The hair loss is basically over the back of the body extending down the dorsum to the base of the tail (Fig. 4–6). It may extend up the tail to the tip, giving the tail a rat-like appearance.

Many of these affected dogs do not have pituitary dwarfism as their only abnormality. It is rare to have an isolated insufficiency of GH. Often there is an insufficiency of other tropic hormones as well. Panhypopituitarism is more common than an isolated insufficiency of GH.

For treatment I have found that administration of 10 international units of bovine GH subcutaneously every other day for 30 days is effective. Following administration of bovine GH, the clinical response of regrowth of the haircoat is seen in approximately four to six weeks (Fig. 4–7).

HYPOSOMATOTROPISM IN THE MATURE ANIMAL

How does one become suspicious of an insufficiency of GH when it begins in the mature animal? In species dependent upon GH for normal glucose homeostasis, an insufficiency may result in hypo-

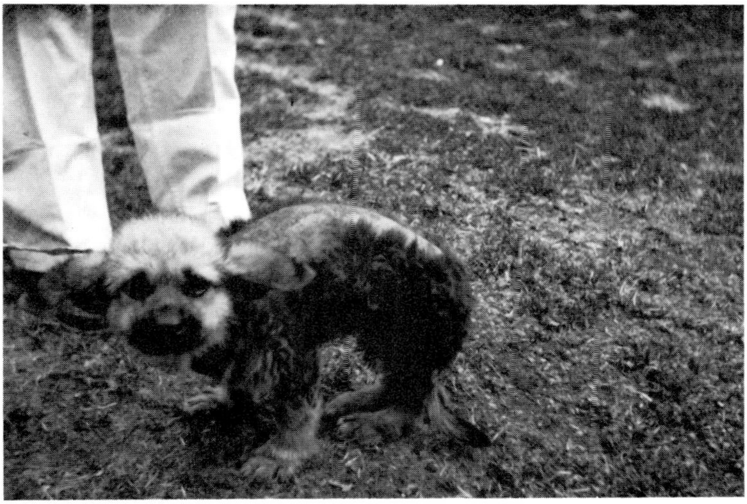

Fig. 4–6. German shepherd pituitary dwarf 3½ years of age. The dwarfism is further complicated by the presence of a chondrodystrophoid-type abnormality of the limbs. Note the loss of hair over the back.

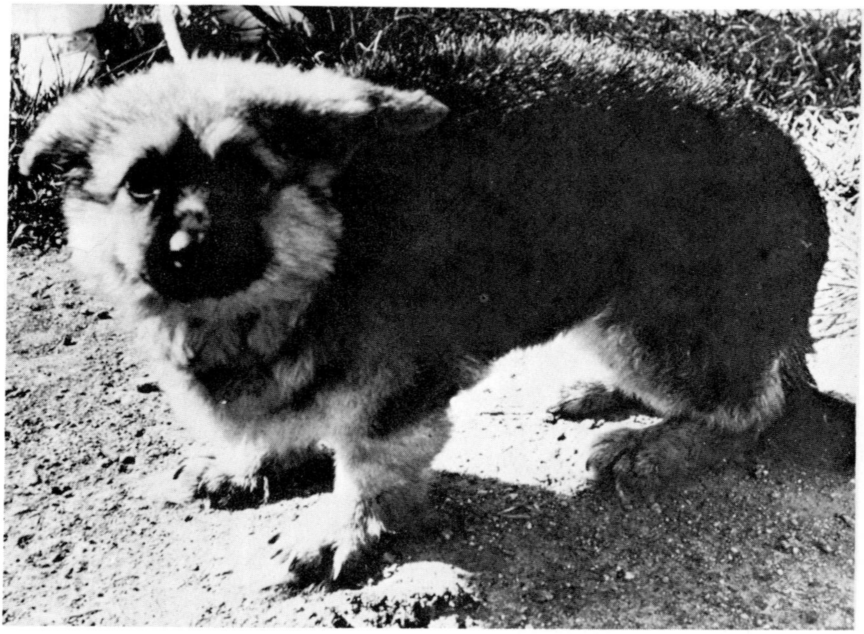

Fig. 4–7. Appearance of German shepherd dwarf shown in Fig. 4–6 after one month of treatment with GH. New hair was evident four weeks after the treatment was discontinued. This photograph was taken six months after therapy.

glycemia. However, the dog maintains a relatively normal glucose level when an insufficiency of growth is present.

There is a disorder in the dog which I have termed "pseudo-Cushing's" syndrome (Fig. 4–8). Animals affected have a hair loss that is visually identical to that of dogs affected with Cushing's syndrome (hyperadrenocorticalism). However, in pseudo-Cushing's syndrome, there are a number of differences from true Cushing's syndrome. First, this disorder occurs in young dogs, usually from two to five years of age. The dogs are in good health except for the hair loss. They lose hair over the trunk and retain hair on the legs and head. In contrast to Cushing's syndrome, there is no pendulous abdomen, polydipsia, polyuria, or lymphopenia. The eosinopenia of Cushing's syndrome is not present, and there is usually a slight to high eosinophil count in the pseudo-Cushing's syndrome. The significance of this latter finding is not obvious. I have treated two of these pseudo-Cushing's syndrome cases with bovine GH. This treatment was attempted after ruling out other endocrine abnormalities. Following treatment with GH, a remarkable response occurred. Hair regrowth was extensive. At the present time there are too few cases to positively define this

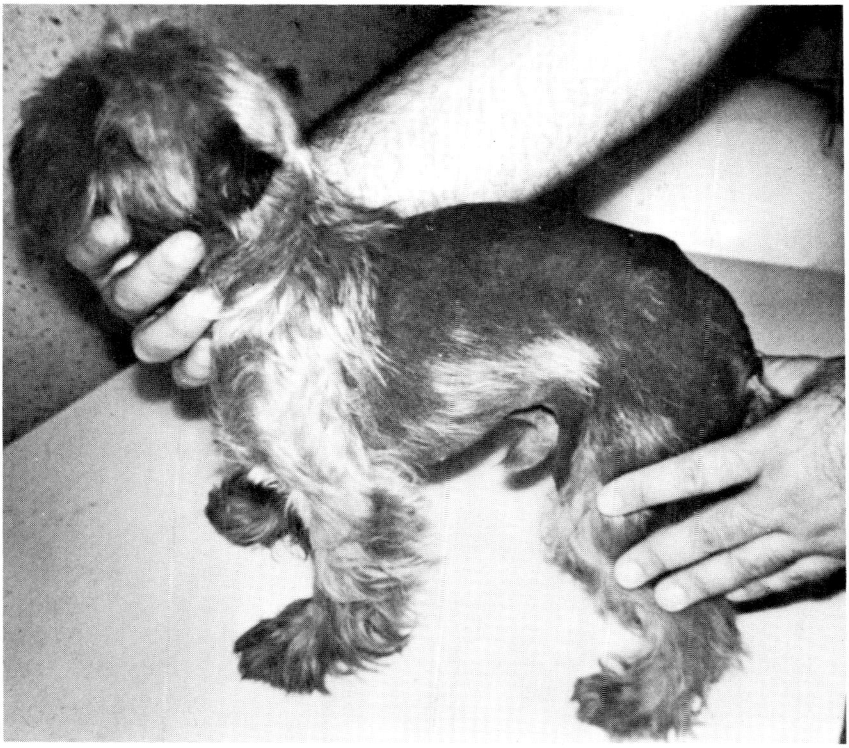

Fig. 4–8. Four-year-old Griffon dog with pseudo-Cushing's syndrome.

abnormality. However, this disorder, which mimics the hair loss of Cushing's syndrome, may be the result of an insufficiency of GH in the adult dog.

HYPOTHYROTROPIC HYPOTHYROIDISM

This disorder is characterized by hypothyroidism that is the result of an insufficiency of thyrotropin (TSH). Clinically it is not yet possible to tell whether there is insufficiency of thyrotropin-releasing factor (TRF) or TSH itself. In the next few years I believe that it will be possible to differentiate exactly which insufficiency is involved.

Clinical signs of hypothyrotropic hypothyroidism are identical to those of primary hypothyroidism; thus, the clinical signs will be further discussed in the chapter on thyroid diseases. In differentiating hypothyrotropic hypothyroidism from primary hypothyroidism, one notes that the thyroid gland is normal in the case of the former; therefore, it responds to the administration of TSH. However, if hypothyrotropic hypothyroidism has been present for a long period of time, the thyroid may be atrophied, and administration of one dose of TSH will not produce the characteristic thyroid response. It is recommended that TSH be given for at least three or four consecutive days to demonstrate whether the thyroid is responsive. One procedure is to administer 10 U of thyrotropin intramuscularly, and quantitate the thyroid response in 24 hours. There is some evidence that the peak secretion of thyroxine following TSH administration occurs within 10 to 12 hours. For demonstration of this maximum response, the sample should be taken earlier than the standard 24-hour test procedure. Serum thyroxine levels before and after TSH should be quantitated by an immunoassay, or by the competitive protein-binding assay, which is modified for the low levels of thyroxine found in dog blood.

Hypothyrotropic hypothyroidism may be associated with other pituitary or hypothalamic dysfunction. Since the treatment of the hypothyrotropic hypothyroidism is identical to that for primary hypothyroidism, it is not necessary to clinically differentiate the two types of hypothyroidism for therapy. If other signs of pituitary or hypothalamic dysfunction are present, it is necessary to differentiate the two types of hypothyroidism. Treatment of hypothyroidism will be discussed in detail in the chapter on the thyroid gland.

HYPOADRENOCORTICOTROPIC ADRENAL INSUFFICIENCY

Hypoadrenocorticotropic or secondary adrenal insufficiency is a disorder rarely diagnosed in the dog. The reason is that clinical signs are not evident in most cases. The dog is able to function adequately with decreased or absent levels of ACTH, and also with decreased levels of glucocorticoids. It has been my experience to diagnose hypoadrenocorticotropic adrenal insufficiency when evidence of other pituitary dysfunction is present, such as in pituitary dwarfism. Hematologic changes suggest the insufficiency of glucocorticoids, i.e., eosinophilia and lymphocytosis. Differential white blood counts may show the eosinophils to be as high as 15 to 20%. Although the affected animals usually are asymptomatic, they may demonstrate more definite signs of adrenal insufficiency when under exceptional stress. Based on this fact, if hypoadrenocorticotropic adrenal insufficiency is diagnosed, it is practical to protect the dog by instituting glucocorticoid replacement therapy, such as 2.5 to 5 mg of cortisol per os daily.

HYPOGONADOTROPIC HYPOGONADISM

Hypogonadotropic hypogonadism is rarely documented in the dog. Because of the unavailability of specific clinical assay procedures for canine FSH and LH, this diagnosis is based on the clinical signs and response to therapy. When clinical signs of hypogonadism are present in the young animal, whether in a young bitch that has never come into estrus or in the male with poor testicular development, the tentative diagnosis is reasonable. Unfortunately, at times the diagnosis of this disorder is only made in retrospect — after a therapeutic regime of gonadotropins has been corrective.

One therapeutic technique utilized in the bitch is the administration of compounds with FSH (pregnant mare serum) at the rate of 50 IU per pound of body weight up to a maximum of 1500 U. This dose is repeated at weekly intervals, for a maximum of three treatments. If the dog comes into standing estrus during treatment, it is additionally treated, within 48 hours of standing estrus, with a drug containing LH (chorionic gonadotropin) at the same dosage rate as for the FSH preparation. The owner is instructed to attempt breeding the animal every other day until the bitch refuses to accept the male.

Recently in human medicine, some insufficiencies of gonadotropins have been successfully treated with clomiphene citrate (Clomid). This drug increases the release of gonadotropins by the anterior pituitary gland. Since it has been used in only a small number of dogs, its effectiveness for therapy of hypogonadism in the dog is not known.

PANHYPOPITUITARISM

An insufficiency of all the anterior pituitary hormones is called panhypopituitarism. My clinical impression is that canine panhypopituitarism occurs more commonly than the isolated pituitary hormone insufficiency. Accordingly, whenever a diagnosis of pituitary dwarfism is made, the possibility of panhypopituitarism should be considered. Evaluation of thyroid, adrenal, and gonad function should be determined. Of all the cases of panhypopituitarism that I have seen, I have found the condition to be more common in German shepherds than in other breeds. When a diagnosis of panhypopituitarism is made, treatment of the hypothyroidism and the adrenal insufficiency is necessary to maintain the animal in good health. The gonad dysfunction can also be treated if the owner requests it When GH becomes more available, the haircoat may be maintained in satisfactory condition.

SELECTED READING

1. Argires, J. P. and Nelson, J.: Pituitary apoplexy: review of the literature and two case reports. South. Med. J., *59*:785, 1966.
2. Dandy, W. E., and Reichert, F. L. Studies on experimental hypophysectomy in dogs. III. Somatic, mental and glandular effects. Bull. Johns Hopkins Hosp., *62*:122, 1938.
3. Espiner, E. A., and Donald, R. A.: Pituitary and gonadal function in hypogonadotrophic hypogonadism. Acta Endocrinol., *73*:209, 1973.
4. Fredrickson, D. S., Ganong, W. F., and Hume, D. M.: Thyroid uptake of radioactive iodine in the dog; effect of diet, hypophysectomy, and TSH. Proc. Soc. Exp. Biol. Med., *89*:416, 1955.

5. Ganong, W. F., Pemberton, D. L., and Van Brunt, E. E.: Adrenocortical responsiveness to ACTH and angiotensin, II. In hypophysectomized dogs and dogs treated with large doses of glucocorticoids. Endocrinology, *81*:1147, 1967.
6. Goodman, H. G., Grumbach, M. M., and Kaplan, S. L.: Growth and growth hormone. II. A comparison of isolated growth hormone deficiency and multiple pituitary hormone deficiencies in 35 patients with idiopathic hypopituitary dwarfism. N. Engl. J. Med., *278*:57, 1968.
7. Haddock, L., Vega, L. A., Aguilo, F., and Rodriguez, O.: Adrenocortical, thyroidal and human growth hormone reserve in Sheehan's syndrome. Johns Hopkins Med. J., *131*:80, 1972.
8. Heap, R. B., Holzbauer, M., and Newport, H. M.: Adrenal secretion rates of C-19 and C-21 steroids before and after hypophysectomy in the pig and the dog. J. Endocrinol., *36*:159, 1966.
9. Kinsella, R. A., Mueheims, G. H., and Francis, F. E.: Adrenal response to hypophysectomy in the newborn dog. Proc. Soc. Exp. Biol. Med., *131*:1389, 1969.
10. Kirkland, R. T., Kirkland, J. L., Librik, L., and Clayton, G. W.: Results of intermittent human growth hormone (hGH) therapy in hypopituitary dwarfism. J. Clin. Endocrinol. Metab., *37*:204, 1973.
11. Martin, F. I. R.: Pituitary deficiency in patients with pituitary tumours. Australas. Ann. Med., *15*:40, 1966.
12. Monos, E., Edit, K., and Kovach, A. G. B.: Adrenal blood flow and corticosteroid secretion: I. The acute effect of hypophysectomy on adrenal blood flow and corticohormone secretion in the anaesthetized dog. Acta Physiol. (Hungary), *28*:139, 1965.
13. Murdoch, R.: Sheehan's syndrome. Lancet, *1*:1327, 1962.
14. Patel, Y. C., and Kilpatrick, J. A.: Pituitary enlargement with longstanding myxoedema. N. Z. Med. J., *70*:21, 1969.
15. Plager, J. E., Bray, G. A., and Jackson, J. E.: Pituitary-ACTH response to metopirone and endotoxin administration in the dog. Endocrinology, *72*:876, 1963.
16. Rabkin, M. T., and Frantz, A. G.: Hypopituitarism: a study of growth hormone and other endocrine functions. Ann. Intern. Med., *64*:1197, 1966.
17. Renauld, A., Pinto, J. E. B., Sverdilk, R. C., Florin, A., and Follia, V.: Studies on the effect of combined growth hormone and cortisol on the insulin response to glucose in the hypophysectomized dog. Horm. Metab. Res., *3*:6, 1971.
18. Rimoin, D. L., et al.: Growth hormone in African pygmies. Lancet, *2*:523, 1967.
19. Rimoin, D. L., Merimee, T. J., and McKusick, V. A.: Growth-hormone deficiency in man: an isolated recessively inherited defect. Science, *152*:1635, 1966.
20. Sirek, A., Schoeffling, K., Webster, M., and Sirek, O. V.: Absence of effect of bovine growth hormone on blood sugar of Houssay dogs. Can. J. Physiol. Pharmacol., *42*:299, 1964.
21. Soyka, L. F., Bode, H. H., Crawford, J. D., and Flynn, F. J., Jr.: Effectiveness of long-term human growth hormone therapy for short stature in children with growth hormone deficiency. J. Clin. Endocrinol. Metab., *30*:1, 1970.
22. Takeda, Y.: Hormonal effects on distribution and excretion of iodide-I^{131} in the dog. Am. J. Physiol., *206*:1237, 1964.
23. Tiscornia, O. M., and Dreiling, D. A.: Microsurgical ablation of the canine pituitary gland. Surgery, *60*:1077, 1966.
24. Underwood, L. E., Voina, S. J., and Van Wyk, J. J.: Restoration of growth by human growth hormone (Roos) in hypopituitary dwarfs immunized by other human growth hormone preparations: clinical and immunological studies. J. Clin. Endocrinol. Metab., *38*:288, 1974.
25. Updike, G. B., Jr., and Corey, E. L.: Experimental attempts to produce anterior pituitary necrosis in the rat and dog. Am. J. Obstet. Gynecol., *90*:25, 1964.
26. Woolf, P. D., and Schalch, D. S.: Hypopituitarism secondary to hypothalamic insufficiency. Ann. Intern. Med., *78*:88, 1973.
27. Zukoski, C. F., and Ney, R. L.: ACTH secretion after pituitary stalk secretion in the dog. Am. J. Physiol., *211*:851, 1966.

Chapter

5

Hyperfunction of the Anterior Pituitary Gland

Abnormalities that result from a hypersecretion of one or more of the anterior pituitary hormones have rarely been reported. To my knowledge, thyrotoxicosis associated with a pituitary tumor that is secreting excess thyrotropin has not been described in the dog. Although there is suspicion that certain ovarian and testicular disorders are associated with altered secretions of gonadotropins, definite evidence is absent. Excessive secretion of ACTH causing canine Cushing's disease (hyperadrenocorticalism) has been described numerous times. However, its incidence in the canine population may have been overstated in the past. While a certain percentage of cases of hyperadrenocorticalism are due to pituitary tumors (Cushing's disease), it is my experience that only about 10% are the result of pituitary-ACTH-producing tumors.

In some of the older literature it appeared that a large percentage of cases of hyperadrenocorticalism were usually associated with pituitary neoplasia. This apparent bias was created by some authors reporting all patients with pituitary tumors in which clinical signs of hyperadrenocorticalism existed. Utilizing this type of analysis, all of these cases had functioning pituitary tumors. However, in recent work in which hyperadrenocorticalism was documented using steroid assays, careful examination of the pituitary glands during necropsy demonstrated that only a small percentage, no more than 10 or 15%, were the result of a functioning pituitary tumor.

Acidophilic adenomas or adenocarcinomas of the pituitary gland that secrete excessive amounts of GH have rarely been reported. However, there is no implication that this abnormality is as uncommon as reported. Polymorphism in the dog creates difficulty in diagnosing a disease produced by the hypersecretion of GH (hypersomatotropism). Excessive secretion of GH in a mixed-breed dog would be very difficult to ascertain based on changes in conformation.

GIGANTISM

Pituitary gigantism is the disorder resulting in overall increase in size due to excessive secretion of GH during the growing phase of the animal and before epiphyseal closure. Hypersomatotropism, present when the epiphyses are open, results in an increased longitudinal growth of long bones. An increase in stature and size occurs in the affected animal. Information on pituitary gigantism in the dog is based on experimental studies following administration of GH. Reports on spontaneous pituitary gigantism in the canine population are practically nonexistent. Based upon experimental data, excessive GH administered to the growing dog produces gigantism (Fig. 5–1). However, the degree of gigantism is dependent upon the breed of dog affected. Dogs with "normal-type" limbs, i.e., the German shepherd type, will develop the expected pituitary gigantism. If excessive GH is administered to a chondrodysplastic dog, the results will be different. The longitudinal growth in the limb bones of the dachshund is affected only slightly, if at all (Fig. 5–2). Since the chondrodysplastic limb is not affected significantly by GH, there is little increase in

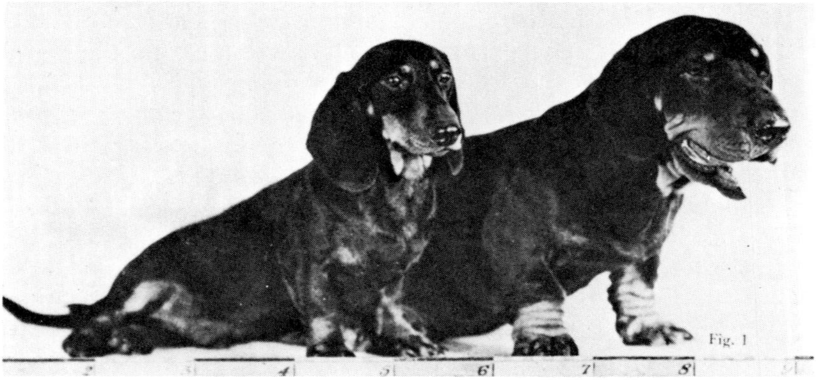

Fig. 5–1. Changes produced in the dachshund by the experimental administration of GH; the untreated littermate (left) and the treated dog (right). The latter was treated daily for six months with intraperitoneal injections of bovine GH. (From Evans, H. M., et al.: Memoirs of Univ. of Calif., II, 1933. Originally published by the University of California Press; reprinted by permission of The Regents of the University of California.)

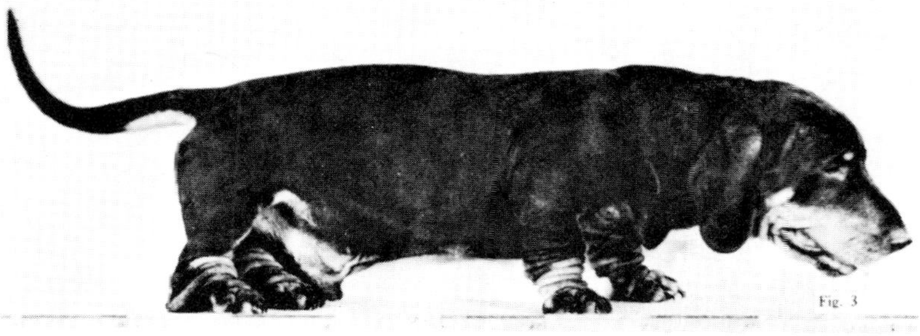

Fig. 5–2. Close-up of the dachshund treated with excessive GH shown in Fig. 5–1. Note that although there is a great increase in the size of the dog, the chondrodysplastic limbs are unaffected. (From Evans, H. M., et al.: Memoirs of Univ. of Calif. II, 1933. Originally published by the University of California Press; reprinted by permission of The Regents of the University of California.)

height. In response to excessive GH, the dachshund spine elongates proportionally more than do long bones. Therefore, excessive GH during the growing period results in a longer dachshund, rather than a taller one.

Based upon the fact that the dog readily develops diabetes mellitus with hypersomatotropism, one might expect the giant breed of dog to have a higher incidence of diabetes. This conclusion has not been verified clinically. One possible explanation is that the canine models of diabetes mellitus due to excessive GH administration have been produced by utilizing bovine GH. It may not be true that a high incidence of diabetes mellitus secondary to an excessive secretion of endogenous GH would occur naturally. According to a report in the literature, one dog has developed diabetes mellitus secondary to hypersomatotropism.

Although pituitary gigantism has rarely been diagnosed in the dog, veterinarians are often asked to examine a dog that has characteristics other than those of a purebred dog. Even if the breeding history suggests that the dog is a purebred, the veterinarian often dismisses the case as an example of superfecundation because he assumes that the breeding history is not as accurate as that presented by the owner. It is possible that some of these animals with altered characteristics may have abnormal secretion of GH. This description of canine pituitary gigantism is intended to alert the veterinarian to the possibility of the existence of this disorder. When a readily available assay for canine GH becomes a reality, more pituitary giants will be described.

The pituitary lesion associated with gigantism is usually the acidophilic tumor, or hyperplasia of the acidophils. As more evidence is gained with this disorder, there will probably be a finding of pituitary tissue that is normal morphologically and histologically.

ACROMEGALY

Excessive secretion of GH after epiphyseal closure will not stimulate longitudinal growth of bones. Consequently, there is an increase in appositional growth of bone. This abnormality increases the size of many features or characteristics of the animal. In man the term acromegaly denotes enlargement of terminal points (or acra), such as the jaws, feet, nose, and hands. Acromegaly in the dog has rarely been described (Fig. 5–3). The infrequent description of this disease in the veterinary literature is probably based upon the profession's unawareness of this disorder, rather than its apparent rarity.

There are other aspects of hypersomatotropism that are important. If the abnormality is present in the growing individual, as stated previously, he becomes a pituitary giant. However, if the disorder continues after epiphyseal closure, the individual will also be acromegalic. Experimentally it has been shown that there is not only the change in longitudinal and appositional bone growth, but also there is general enlargement of all tissues throughout the body. The skin is thickened, which often produces large fold-like structures in the skin. The thickened skin associated with acromegaly appears different from the thickened skin common to other endocrine abnormalities. With hypersomatotropism, the animal has a good haircoat, which is described as shiny and glossy. In contrast with canine hypothyroidism, the skin is thickened and the haircoat is poor, i.e., dull and easily epilated.

In one reported diabetic dog, suspected to be diabetic secondary to acromegaly, 100 U of protamine zinc insulin had to be administered twice daily to stabilize the diabetes. In addition to the insulin insensitivity, acromegalic features developed (Fig. 5–4). At necropsy, eosinophilic hyperplasia of the anterior pituitary gland was observed. Therapy of pituitary gigantism and/or acromegaly has not been carried out in the dog. Therapeutically in man, acidophilic tumors are relatively sensitive to x-ray irradiation. It is impossible to predict whether the canine pituitary would be as responsive to x-ray irradiation as is man's.

With all hypersecreting abnormalities of the anterior pituitary gland, if the dysfunction is related to an expanding lesion, there may also be clinical signs referable to the central nervous system. Signs of diminishing vision are difficult to recognize in the dog with an enlarging pituitary tumor. When visual disturbances are recognized,

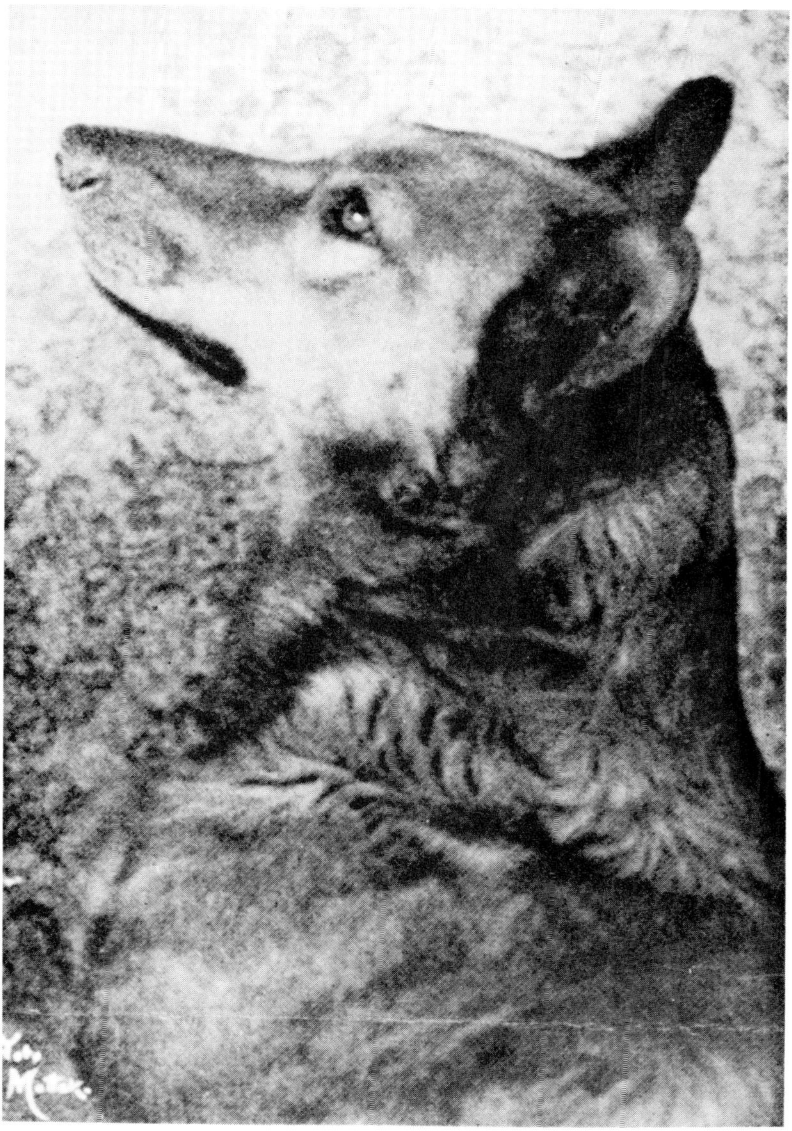

Fig. 5–3. Photograph of 6-year-old Malines shepherd dog prior to development of acromegalic features. The typical sharp features of the head are present. (From Groen, J. J., Frenkel, H. S., and Offerhaus, L.: Diabetes, *13*:493, 1964.)

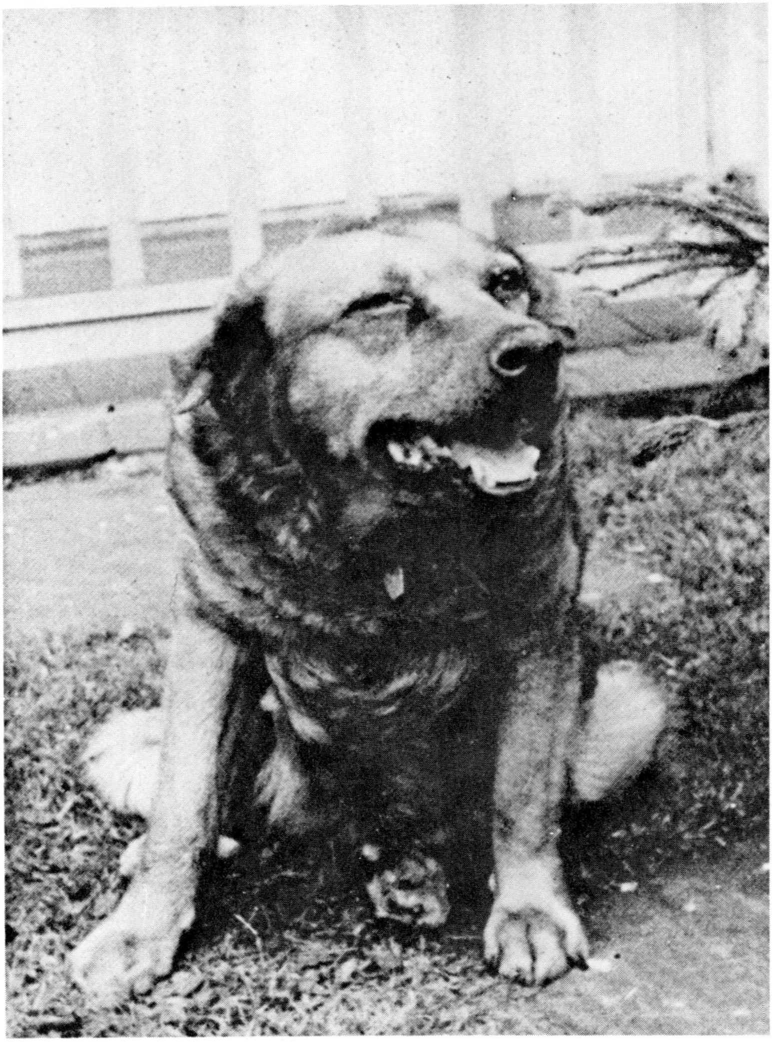

Fig. 5–4. The Malines shepherd dog shown in Fig. 5–3 after the development of acromegalic features. The head had become blunt, the jaws conspicuously heavy, and the skin thickened. (From Groen, J. J., Frenkel, H. S., and Offerhaus, L.: Diabetes, *13*:494, 1964.)

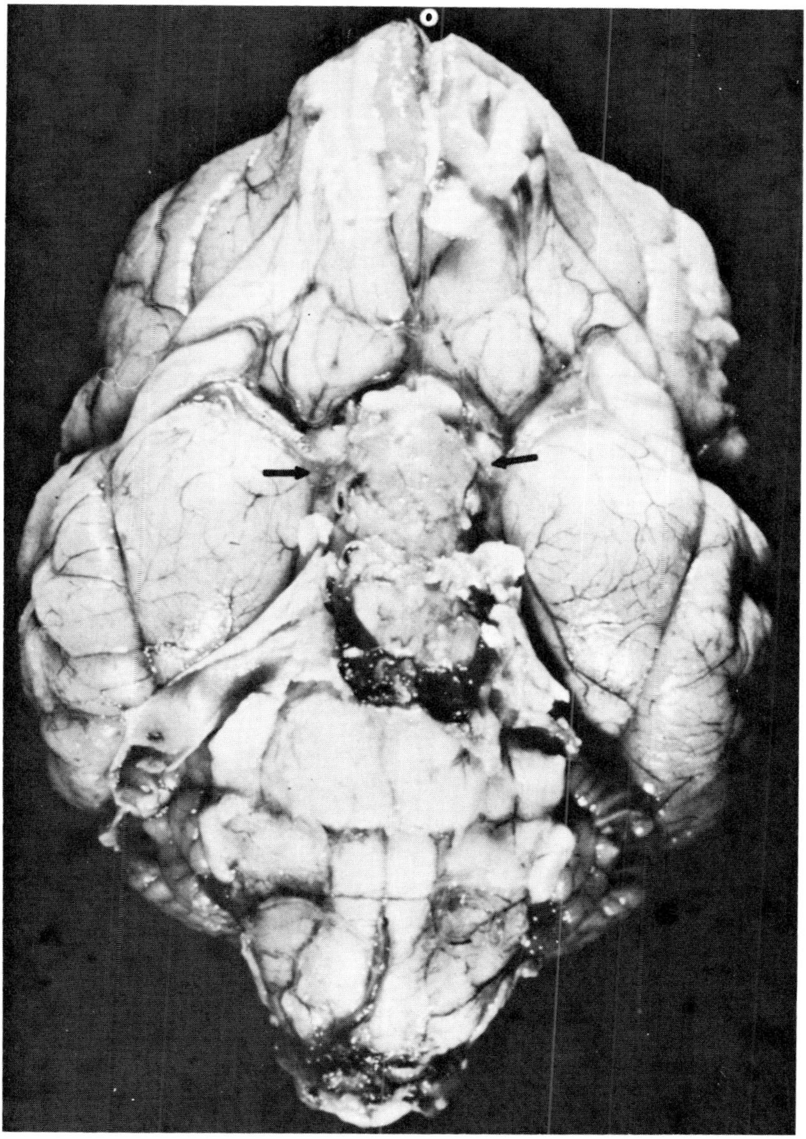

Fig. 5–5. Pituitary chromophobe adenoma. Ventral view showing an oval mass extending from the optic chiasm to the anterior pons. (From Schwartzman, R M., and Fegley, H.: J. Am. Vet. Med. Assoc., *147*:649, 1965.)

they usually are associated with relatively large tumors. There are several possibilities that might explain how this condition differs from that in man. The optic chiasma is more craniad and slightly further separated from the pituitary in the dog. Also, the bony sella turcica that encompasses the canine pituitary gland is less complete than that in man. In the dog any enlarging pituitary mass can expand in most positions around the circumference of the pituitary gland. Man has a "weakened" area craniad to the pituitary. Expanding pituitary lesions in man more easily infringe on the optic chiasma. If the pituitary lesion is large enough to encroach into the hypothalamus and create an increase in intracranial pressure, other neurologic abnormalities may also be present.

CUSHING'S DISEASE

Dr. Harvey Cushing first described the abnormality associated with hyperfunction of the adrenal cortex in a person who had a basophilic

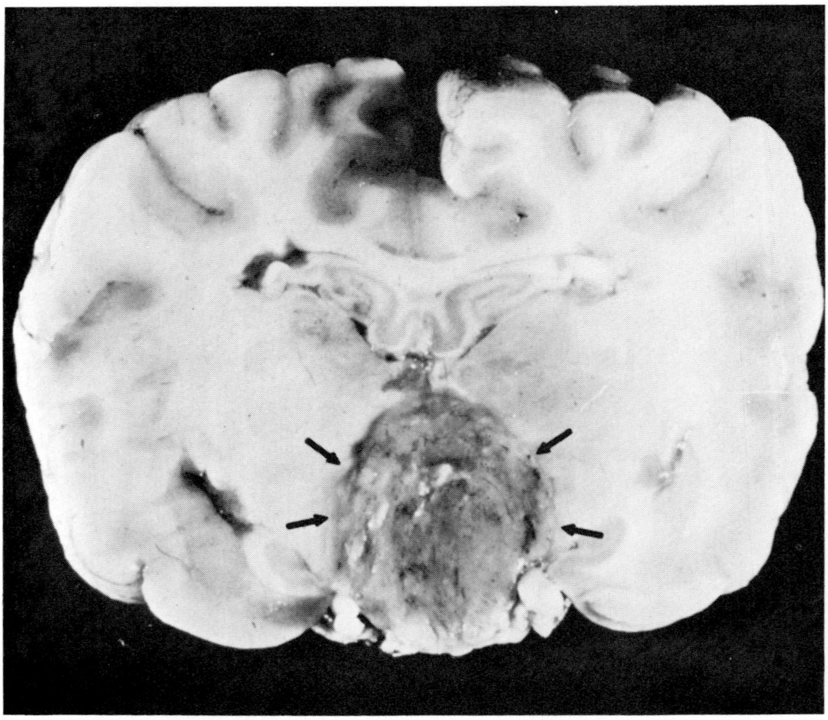

Fig. 5–6. Cross section of the chromophobe adenoma shown in Fig. 5–5. The tumor had grown dorsally and involved the hypothalamus and thalamus. (From Schwartzman, R. M., and Fegley, H.: J. Am. Vet. Med. Assoc., *147*:649, 1965.)

adenoma of the pituitary gland. The term Cushing's disease has come to signify the abnormality of hyperadrenocorticalism associated with a tumor of the anterior pituitary gland. These basophilic tumors were thought to secrete excessive amounts of ACTH. Now with sensitive assay procedures for ACTH, it has been determined that the basophilic tumor is not usually a hypersecretor of ACTH. The chromophobic tumors appear to be ACTH secreting tumors. The abnormality, Cushing's syndrome, is hyperadrenocorticalism caused by any abnormality other than a functional pituitary tumor. It is unusual in the dog for the pituitary lesion to cause neurologic or visual disturbances. Canine pituitary tumors producing Cushing's disease are relatively slow-growing neoplasms. Only the rapidly growing, large pituitary tumors produce associated neurologic signs (Figs. 5–5, 5–6, and 5–7).

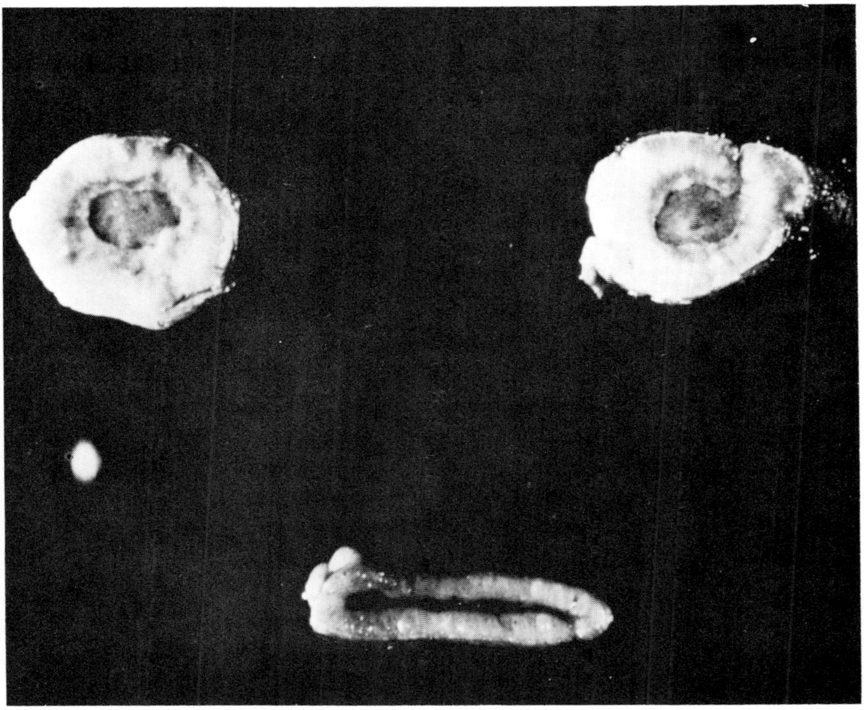

Fig. 5–7. Bilateral adrenocortical hyperplasia. Cross section of affected adrenals (above) from the dog with the functioning pituitary chromophobe adenoma shown in Fig. 5–5. The adrenal glands are rounded, and the cortex thickened. A normal adrenal gland is shown below. (From Schwartzman, R. M., and Fegley, H.: J. Am. Vet. Med. Assoc., *147*:648, 1965.)

Treatment of Cushing's disease using either irradiation or surgical removal of the offending tumor has limited value in the dog. Since most of these tumors are slow growing, bilateral adrenalectomy completely ameliorates the clinical signs. With proper maintenance therapy, it may be many years before the pituitary tumor becomes large enough to cause any further disturbance.

SELECTED READING

1. Capen, C. C., and Koestner, A.: Functional chromophobe adenomas of the canine adenohypophysis. Pathol. Vet., *4*:326, 1967.
2. Capen, C. C., Martin, S. L., and Koestner, A.: Neoplasms in the adenohypophysis of dogs. Pathol. Vet., *4*:301, 1967.
3. Capen, C. C., Martin, S. L., and Koestner, A.: The ultrastructure and histopathology of an acidophil adenoma of the canine adenohypophysis. Pathol. Vet., *4*:348, 1967.
4. Cushing, H.: The basophil adenomas of the pituitary body and their clinical manifestations. (Pituitary basophilism). Bull. Johns Hopkins Hosp., *50*:137, 1932.
5. Edmonds, M. W., Simpson, W. J. K., and Meakin, J. W.: External irradiation of the hypophysis for Cushing's disease. Can. Med. Assoc. J., *107*:860, 1972.
6. Evans, H. M., et al.: The Growth and Gonad-Stimulating Hormones of the Anterior Hypophysis. Memoirs of the Univ. of Calif., Vol. II. Univ. of Calif. Press, Berkeley, 1933.
7. Gilbert, G. J., and Willey, E. N.: Pituitary chromophobe adenoma in the bulldog. J. Am. Vet. Med. Assoc., *154*:1071, 1969.
8. Groen, J. J., Frenkel, H. S., and Offerhaus, L.: Observations on a case of spontaneous diabetes mellitus in a dog. Diabetes, *13*:492, 1964.
9. Hottendorf, G. H., Nielsen, S. W., and Liberman, L. L.: Acidophil adenoma of the pituitary gland and other neoplasms in a boxer. J. Am. Vet. Med. Assoc., *148*:1046, 1966.
10. Hunder, G. G.: Pathogenesis of Cushing's disease. Mayo Clin. Proc., *41*:29, 1966.
11. King, J. M., Kavanaugh, J. F., and Bentinck-Smith, J.: Diabetes mellitus with pituitary neoplasms in a horse and a dog. Cornell Vet., *52*:133, 1962.
12. Meier, H.: Etiologic considerations of spontaneous tumors in animals with special reference to the endocrine system. Ann. N. Y. Acad. Sci., *108*:881, 1963.
13. Molinatti, G. M., Camanni, F., Massara, F., and Messina, M.: Implantation of the sella turcica with ^{90}yttrium in the treatment of Cushing's syndrome of pituitary origin. J. Clin. Endocrinol. Metab., *27*:861, 1967.
14. Rijnberk, A., Der Kinderen, P. J., and Thijssen, J. H. H.: Canine Cushing's syndrome. Zentralbl. Veterinaermed., *16*:13, 1969.
15. Robinson, J. L.: Sudden blindness with pituitary tumors. J. Neurosurg., *36*:83, 1972.
16. Rovit, R. L., and Duane, T. D.: Cushing's syndrome and pituitary tumors. Am. J. Med., *46*:416, 1969.
17. Schwartzman, R. M., and Fegley, H.: Clinico-path. conference, Univ. of Penna., Sch. of Vet. Med., J. Am. Vet. Med. Assoc., *147*:642, 1965.
18. Young, D. G., Bahn, R. C., and Randall, R. V.: Pituitary tumors associated with acromegaly. J. Clin. Endocrinol. Metab., *25*:249, 1965.

Chapter 6

The Posterior Pituitary Gland

ANATOMY

The posterior pituitary gland (neurohypophysis) is composed of the median eminence, the infundibular stem, and the infundibular process (posterior lobe). The posterior pituitary lobe is the termination of neurons that have cell bodies originating in the hypothalamus. There are two nuclei in the hypothalamus where cell bodies send their axons to the infundibular stem and into the posterior pituitary lobe itself. These two are the supraoptic nucleus and the paraventricular nucleus. Unmyelinated fibers originating from these nuclei are joined with fibers of the tuberohypophyseal tract to form the hypothalamohypophyseal tract, which terminates in the posterior lobe of the pituitary.

HISTOLOGY

The chief cellular component of the posterior pituitary is the pituicyte. It is essentially a central nervous system connective tissue cell or neuroglia cell. In addition to these cells, the posterior pituitary comprises unmyelinated nerve fibers and their nerve endings. The histologic composition of the posterior pituitary gland reflects its embryologic derivation from the floor of the diencephalon.

PHYSIOLOGY

The supraoptic and paraventricular nuclei function as osmoreceptors. The supraoptic nucleus is more important in this role. An increase in plasma osmolality stimulates the cells in the nuclei to synthesize vasopressin (antidiuretic hormone, ADH), which is transmitted via the axon to be released in the posterior lobe. ADH circulates in plasma without significant binding to serum proteins.

The kidney and liver are the major sites of ADH deactivation. Approximately 10% of ADH, depending on the species, is excreted in the free form in the urine. ADH is important in maintaining a stable serum osmolality by effecting a controlled water excretion. Its major antidiuretic effect results from its ability to alter the reabsorption of water in the distal convoluted tubule and the collecting ducts of the kidney. This action is mainly initiated by increasing the permeability of these renal areas to water.

In mammals there are two active posterior pituitary hormones, vasopressin (ADH) and oxytocin. The latter is secreted mainly by the paraventricular nucleus. Of the two chemical forms of vasopressin in mammals (Fig. 6–1), the most common is arginine vasopressin, which is secreted by most mammals. Lysine vasopressin is present in the pig, the hippopotamus, and other closely related species. In the dog, lysine vasopressin has little activity when compared to its native form, arginine vasopressin. Although the antidiuretic activity resides mainly in vasopressin, oxytocin, being similar in chemical structure, has some overlapping activity. Oxytocin has slight antidiuretic activity, and vasopressin has slight milk ejection activity.

Whenever there is an increased plasma osmolality, the supraoptic nucleus responds by producing ADH. The hormone descends by way of the nerve fibers and is picked up by the capillaries in the posterior pituitary. From there it is transported to its target cells in the kidney where it stimulates the reabsorption of water in the distal convoluted tubule along with actively reabsorbed salt. Aldosterone acts as a permissive hormone for ADH action, in that small amounts of aldosterone appear to be necessary for maximum antidiuresis.

CYS – TYR – **PHE** – GLU(NH_2) – ASP(NH_2) – CYS – PRO – **ARG** – GLY(NH_2)
1 2 3 4 5 6 7 8 9

8–ARGININE VASOPRESSIN

CYS – TYR – **PHE** – GLU(NH_2) – ASP(NH_2) – CYS – PRO – **LYS** – GLY(NH_2)

8–LYSINE VASOPRESSIN

CYS – TYR – **ILEU** – GLU(NH_2) – ASP(NH_2) – CYS – PRO – **LEU** – GLY(NH_2)

OXYTOCIN

Fig. 6–1. Structures of mammalian neurohypophyseal hormones. Differences in peptide chains are noted in bold lettering. (From Sawin, C. T.: Little, Brown & Co., Inc., 1969.)

Oxytocin secretion is mainly stimulated by afferent nerve impulses from a number of sources. Vaginal stimulation or cervical dilatation results in afferent impulses that stimulate the paraventricular nucleus of the hypothalamus to secrete oxytocin. Suckling or manipulation of the nipples has a similar effect. The oxytocin migrates along the nerve fibers and is picked up by capillaries in the posterior pituitary lobe. Oxytocin produces milk expulsion in the breast that is engorged. This hormone also stimulates contraction of the uterus under specific conditions. This latter action occurs physiologically at a specific time during labor. The uterus must be "hormonally" prepared before oxytocin stimulates contractions. Oxytocin produced in the hypothalamus is also carried by the primary venous plexus of the portal system to the anterior pituitary where it stimulates the output of prolactin. Milk production in the endocrinologically prepared breast is stimulated by prolactin.

ROLE OF ADH IN DIABETES INSIPIDUS

Diabetes insipidus is a disease characterized by the excretion of voluminous amounts of urine, sugar free and quite dilute. This disorder can result from destructive lesions of the supraoptic nucleus, the supraoptic-hypophyseal tract, or the posterior pituitary lobe. An insufficiency of ADH decreases reabsorption of water in the distal convoluted tubule and collecting ducts, resulting in an increase in the amount of urine excreted.

ROLE OF OTHER HORMONES IN DIABETES INSIPIDUS

The fact that other hormones are involved in the full expression of diabetes insipidus has been well known for years. Clinically, diabetes insipidus is more severe when there is a functioning anterior pituitary gland. If both the anterior pituitary gland and the posterior pituitary lobe are destroyed, less urine is excreted. In addition, complete hypophysectomy in the experimental animal produces a diabetes insipidus that is less severe than if the posterior pituitary lobe only is removed or destroyed. Clinicians have noted that, in documented cases of diabetes insipidus, clinical signs of water consumption and urine output ameliorate if the anterior pituitary gland is also destroyed.

The significance of other hormones in the genesis of diabetes insipidus is that those produced by the anterior pituitary gland have an effect that is opposite that of ADH. ACTH stimulation of corticosteroid biosynthesis produces diuresis mainly by increasing the glomerular filtration rate. Other data suggest that the corticosteroids inhibit the action of ADH directly in the distal kidney tubule and collecting ducts. It is easy to appreciate that, if an insufficiency of ADH were present, there would be less reabsorption of water in the kidney and an increase in the amount of urine produced. However, if there exists, in addition, an insufficiency of corticosteroids, it would decrease the diuresis. Destruction of the anterior pituitary gland results in less urine production, and accordingly less water consumption. Clinically, if a case of diabetes insipidus is confirmed, and if the amount of water diuresis is decreasing, these circumstances do not necessarily suggest that the disorder is improving. It usually is associated with an expanding lesion of the pituitary gland, which initially damages the posterior lobe or pituitary stalk, and then destroys the anterior pituitary gland. Thus, amelioration of clinical signs of diabetes insipidus may be the forewarning of an expanding pituitary lesion.

In addition to the diuretic action of the corticosteroids, the thyroid hormones produce a similar effect. Therefore, in the completely hypophysectomized animal, or in the spontaneous cases of diabetes insipidus with destruction of the anterior pituitary lobe, an insufficiency of TSH and ACTH are both factors in decreasing the severity of the diabetes insipidus. Support for the role of the thyroid and the adrenal cortex in diabetes insipidus comes from the fact that surgical removal of the thyroid gland decreases the severity of diabetes insipidus. In addition, administration of thyroxine increases water consumption and urine volume in these patients. Bilateral adrenalectomy also decreases the clinical signs of diabetes insipidus, and corticosteroid administration exacerbates the condition.

HYPOFUNCTION OF THE NEUROHYPOPHYSIS — DIABETES INSIPIDUS

Clinical Signs

Diabetes insipidus is a disorder in which the animal produces a large amount of dilute urine with corresponding increased water intake. If complicating factors are not present, the only manifest clinical signs are the polyuria and polydipsia. The amount of urine excreted in the affected dog can be as high as a liter or more, depending upon the size of the dog. The 30- to 40-pound dog with diabetes insipidus usually has a urine volume greater than a liter. Urine volumes as high as five liters are common in the medium to large dog affected with this disorder.

The urine is dilute, and the specific gravity usually is 1.004 or less, depending upon the severity of the diabetes insipidus. In the early stages of the disease, the specific gravity is often higher, but as the disease progresses, it decreases. More accurate than specific gravity in determining the renal concentrating capacity is urine osmolality. With diabetes insipidus the urine osmolality is often as low as 50 to 200 mOsm/kg of water. Urine osmolality is lower than plasma osmolality.

Utilizing a water deprivation test, the urine osmolality usually increases to some extent; however, it cannot become higher than plasma osmolality in the complete absence of ADH.

Etiology

Diabetes insipidus can result from destructive lesions of the supraoptic nucleus in the hypothalamus, the supraoptic-hypophyseal tract, or the posterior pituitary lobe itself. Lesions in vital areas, e. g., tumors, may also cause diabetes insipidus. Other destructive or degenerative lesions in these specific locations can cause the disease. However, many cases of diabetes insipidus in the dog seen clinically are idiopathic, since specific lesions cannot be demonstrated at necropsy.

For years the polydipsia and polyuria associated with canine Cushing's syndrome were thought to be caused by diabetes insipidus. This relationship is not true in most cases in the dog since, following adrenalectomy for the treatment of Cushing's syndrome, the urine volume and osmolality return to normal.

Diagnosis

Several criteria must be met in arriving at a diagnosis of diabetes insipidus. There must be dilute urine with increased volume, and stimuli that normally increase secretion of ADH and decrease urine volume must not elicit the usual effect. Water deprivation in a dog with diabetes insipidus does not produce a normal urine concentration. Although plasma and urine osmolality determinations may be more meaningful than the urine specific gravity, in most instances the latter value will be accurate enough to establish a diagnosis of diabetes insipidus.

Urine specific gravity is low when diabetes insipidus is present. As time progresses during water deprivation, the urine remains dilute and voluminous. The animal has limited ability to increase the urine concentration. In a small number of cases, there are slight increases in the urine specific gravity, up to the value of 1.010 after 12 to 24 hours of water deprivation. In most cases, however, the specific gravity remains low, and may be less than 1.004. The dog, thus, becomes dehydrated. If the urine specific gravity remains near or below 1.004 following 12 hours of water deprivation, it is inadvisable to continue water deprivation since the developing dehydration can result in shock or death.

If the urine specific gravity does increase slightly in the first 12 hours, I allow the water deprivation test to continue, being careful to monitor the animal closely during the next 12 hours. It is not necessary to withhold water for more than 24 hours since a definitive diagnosis of diabetes insipidus usually can be made after 12 hours in a well-developed case. In these patients the urine specific gravity remains in the 1.001 to 1.005 range. In borderline cases of diabetes insipidus, it may take 24 hours of water deprivation to establish a diagnosis, but the urine concentration will not increase significantly.

A more accurate method in making the diagnosis is to obtain the serum and urine osmolality before and after 12 hours of water deprivation. As serum osmolality increases during water deprivation, ADH secretion is stimulated, and it increases the reabsorption of water by the kidney, resulting in an increased urine osmolality. Therefore, if the urine osmolality rises above the serum osmolality, the diagnosis cannot be diabetes insipidus. Normally serum osmolality is in the range of 290 ± 5 mOsm/kg. In diabetes insipidus the osmolality of the urine may be in the range of 50 and 200 mOsm/kg. Following water deprivation, a slight increase in urine osmolality may occur, but if it becomes greater than serum osmolality, the diagnosis of diabetes insipidus has been excluded.

In addition to the dilute urine and a negative response to water deprivation, those with diabetes insipidus respond to the administration of exogenous ADH. To evaluate response to vasopressin, administer 2 to 5 IU of vasopressin tannate in oil intramuscularly once daily for one to three days. During this test, water should not be given ad lib, but restricted in order that maximal urine concentrating ability can be assessed. A positive response to ADH is not significant unless it has first been demonstrated that the animal is unable to concentrate urine following water deprivation.

Another procedure for assessing whether an animal is able to secrete ADH is to infuse hypertonic saline solution over a number of hours. This solution increases plasma osmolality in the same way as does water deprivation. One evaluates the urine concentration, either the specific gravity or the urine osmolality, before infusion of the hypertonic saline solution and at the end of the infusion. This diagnostic technique is more difficult in the dog than in man, since the patient is not as cooperative.

Prognosis and Treatment

Although response to ADH injections is dramatic in cases of diabetes insipidus, the prognosis in the dog is poor. The most important factor appears to be the route of administration of vasopressin tannate in oil. Since this medication must be administered intramuscularly, a painful injection, the owners are unable to keep the animal cooperative after a few weeks or months. For this reason, treatment is not faithfully continued, and the owners are unable to tolerate the dog urinating in the house.

Some newer treatment techniques in human medicine do not seem to be applicable to the dog. For man there is a synthetic vasopressin that is effective as a nasal spray preparation. When the patient becomes thirsty, he increases the amount of nasal spray medication. I have tried this nasal spray preparation in a limited number of cases of canine diabetes insipidus, and have not found it effective.

Other reported treatments for people are certain diuretics, such as chlorothiazide, and some hypoglycemic agents, such as chlorpropamide. When these compounds are used in cases of diabetes insipidus, they paradoxically cause antidiuresis. A number of detailed studies suggest the mechanism of this action. It appears that, although there is some improvement with chlorothiazide therapy experimentally, it is not as effective as vasopressin; therefore, it is of limited clinical use. The actions of chlorpropamide, in its antidiuretic effects on cases of diabetes insipidus, are somewhat similar to those of vasopressin. However, chlorpropamide therapy also produces hypoglycemia, which is often a complicating factor. This side effect has lessened the clinical value of chlorpropamide. In human medicine attempts to avoid this problem involve utilizing a combination of chlorpropamide and chlorothiazide. The rationale is to use less of each drug, and still produce the desired antidiuresis. In my experience with the dog, this type of therapy has not been effective. At the present time, I feel that the only reliable treatment in the dog is the injection of vasopressin tannate in oil, but the potential difficulty associated with intramuscular injections remains.

INAPPROPRIATE SECRETION OF ANTIDIURETIC HORMONE

Since 1957 it has been recognized that man oversecretes ADH in certain situations. This abnormality has been termed the *syndrome of inappropriate secretion of antidiuretic hormone* (SIADH). To my knowledge this disorder has not been described in the veterinary literature, but veterinarians should be aware of its existence. Although SIADH in man was first described in association with certain malignancies, it has also been seen with certain disorders of the central nervous system and the lung. In many reported cases the cause is unknown. With SIADH there is a hypo-osmolality of the serum. The syndrome has been called "inappropriate" because serum osmolality is low, and the stimulus is to decrease the secretion of ADH.

Another important feature of SIADH is hyponatremia and continued urinary excretion of sodium. This condition produces urine that is hyperosmolar to the serum. This disorder differs from adrenocortical insufficiency in that dehydration occurs in the latter. With SIADH, because of the hypo-osmolar state of the serum, the animal is, if anything, overhydrated. If the presence of hyponatremia leads to a diagnosis of adrenal insufficiency, and if the usual treatment does not give the expected response, the clinician should be alerted to the possibility of SIADH.

The findings that I would expect in the dog with SIADH are weakness and, in extreme cases, a comatose state. Also, since any acute disease with pronounced polyuria may result in hyponatremia, this possibility should be considered. These clinical signs can mimic those of adrenal insufficiency due to the severe hyponatremia.

Once a diagnosis of SIADH has been made, successful treatment of this condition depends on understanding that the extracellular fluid volume has increased. Since the clinical signs are the direct result of excessive retention of water, the correct treatment is fluid restriction in order to induce a normal fluid volume. Unfortunately, although the patient with SIADH is hyponatremic, sodium administration produces only a very transient increase in serum sodium because of the continued loss of sodium by the kidney. The administration of sodium should be considered only when a patient is comatose or convulsive. The use of salt-retaining steroids, such as desoxycorticosterone acetate, is not effective in this disorder. The important therapeutic approach is to correct the primary abnormality, which is overhydration due to the inappropriate secretion of ADH. Recent reports have documented a number of cases of SIADH in man during anesthesia and surgery. Therefore, recognition of this disorder is important.

A further difference between SIADH and adrenal insufficiency, and other causes of hyponatremia, is based on the serum potassium level. In adrenal insufficiency the animal is dehydrated, and the extracellular plasma volume is decreased. The serum potassium level is increased. With SIADH there is an increased extracellular fluid volume, and the serum potassium level is normal to low.

In retrospect, I have probably seen a number of these cases. In the past, they were considered to be rare cases of adrenal insufficiency that were nonresponsive to therapy. It was thought that therapy was begun too late. However, it should be emphasized that, when a suspected adrenal insufficiency occurs with no elevation of the potassium level, SIADH should be considered as an alternative diagnosis to primary adrenal insufficiency.

OXYTOCIN

Specific diseases related to either an insufficiency or hypersecretion of oxytocin have not been well documented. However, since this hormone is often used clinically, its biologic actions should be clearly understood.

Since the chemical structure of oxytocin is similar to that of ADH, they have some overlapping properties. However, oxytocin has a relatively weak antidiuretic action. It is produced primarily in the paraventricular nucleus of the hypothalamus, and similarly to ADH, migrates along the nerve axons and is released in the posterior pituitary. Oxytocin is also secreted into the hypothalamic-pituitary-portal system, and is carried to the anterior pituitary where it stimulates the secretion of prolactin.

A number of neurohumoral reflexes are involved in the secretion of oxytocin. One of these is suckling or manipulation of the nipples. This action produces afferent nerve impulses that reach the hypothalamus and initiate the synthesis of oxytocin. Oxytocin is important in the stimulation of prolactin, which is necessary for milk production in the endocrinologically prepared breast. In addition, oxytocin is the "milk-let-down" hormone. Suckling produces expulsion from the milk-engorged breast. Another pathway involved in the secretion of oxytocin is the afferent nerve impulses to the hypothalamus, initiated by dilatation of the cervix or by stimulation of the vagina. This reflex appears to be involved in parturition. Oxytocin is not the initiator of parturition; however, its concentration increases in the circulation during the birth process. Its importance in the contractile activity of the uterus makes it useful clinically.

Pharmacologically, oxytocin is used in the dog in the latter stage of parturition when the cervix is fully dilated and obstruction to fetal delivery is not present. When the uterus is noncontractile, or the contractions are weaker than necessary for expulsion of the newborn, oxytocin is indicated.

The pharmacologic dose of oxytocin (Pitocin) varies with the size of the dog: the usual recommended dosage is 2 to 5 U injected intramuscularly. When utilizing oxytocin for uterine contraction, the let-down of milk may be used as a bioassay procedure to evaluate the correct dosage of oxytocin. After the injection, allow up to two hours for the response. In many cases, only one injection may be necessary. If the bitch lactates, the dosage of oxytocin is sufficient. If parturition does not proceed at this point, then surgical intervention may be necessary. However, if milk let-down is not evident after two hours, repeat the initial dose of oxytocin, and continue repeating it every two hours until there is either milk let-down or expulsion of the newborn. Precautions must be taken to eliminate any obstruction to fetal expulsion; otherwise, uterine rupture and its accompanying consequences may ensue.

SELECTED READING

1. Andersen, R. N., and Egdahl, R. H.: Effect of vasopressin on pituitary-adrenal secretion in the dog. Endocrinology, *74*:538, 1964.
2. Andreani, D., Cinotti, G. A., and Stirati, G.: Chlorpropamide in idiopathic diabetes insipidus. Metabolism, *18*:874, 1969.
3. Bartter, F. C., and Schwartz, W. B.: The syndrome of inappropriate secretion of antidiuretic hormone. Am. J. Med., *42*:790, 1967.
4. Baisset, A., Lac, D. T., and Montastruc, P.: Action hypoglycemiante de la vasopressine chez le chien surrenalectomise ou hypophysectomise. C. R. Soc. Biol., *157*:877, 1963.

5. Bode, H. H., and Miettinen, O. S.: Nephrogenic diabetes insipidus: absence of close linkage with Xg. Am. J. Hum. Genet., *22*:221, 1970.
6. Brennan, L. A., Bonjour, J. P., and Malvin, R. L.: ADH levels during salt depletion in dogs. Eur. J. Clin. Invest., *2*:43, 1971.
7. Brook, A. H., and Share, L.: On the question of protein binding and the diffusibility of circulating antidiuretic hormone in the dog. Endocrinology, *78*:779, 1966.
8. Burka, E. R.: Renal function in diabetes insipidus. Arch. Intern. Med., *109*:717, 1962.
9. Chien, S., Peric, B., and Usami, S.: The reflex nature of release of antidiuretic hormone upon common carotid occlusion in vagotomized dogs. Proc. Soc. Exp. Biol. Med., *111*:193, 1962.
10. Coggins, C. H., and Leaf, A.: Diabetes insipidus. Am. J. Med., *42*:807, 1967.
11. Davis, B. B., Knox, F. G., and Berliner, R. W.: Effect of vasopressin on proximal tubule sodium reabsorption in the dog. Am. J. Physiol., *212*:1361, 1967.
12. Dingman, J. F., and Hauger-Klevene, J. H.: Treatment of diabetes insipidus: synthetic lysine vasopressin nasal solution. J. Clin. Endocrinol. Metab., *24*:550, 1964.
13. Edwards, C. R. W., Kitau, M. J., Chard, T., and Besser, G. M.: Vasopressin analogue DDAVP in diabetes insipidus: clinical and laboratory studies. Br. Med. J., *18*:375, 1973.
14. Ehrlich, R. M. and Kooh, S. W.: The use of chlorpropamide in diabetes insipidus in children. Pediatrics, *45*:236, 1970.
15. Ettinger, B., and Forsham, P. H.: Mechanism of chlorpropamide antidiuresis in diabetes insipidus. J. Clin. Endocrinol. Metab., *31*:552, 1970.
16. Fang, H. S., Liu, H. M., and Wang, S. C.: Liberation of antidiuretic hormone following hypothalamic stimulation in the dog. Am. J. Physiol., *202*:212, 1962.
17. Fichman, M. P., and Brooker, G.: Deficient renal cyclic adenosine 3′–5′ monophosphate production in nephrogenic diabetes insipidus. J. Clin. Endocrinol. Metab., *35*:35, 1972.
18. Gillenwater, J. Y.: Antidiuretic properties of chlorothiazide in diabetes insipidus dogs. Metabolism, *14*:539, 1965.
19. Greiss, K. C., Moses, A. M., and Krieger, D. T.: Pituitary adenoma associated with inappropriate antidiuretic hormone secretion. Acta Endocrinol., *76*:59, 1974.
20. Grieg, W. A.: Diabetes insipidus in the dog and cat. Proc. 17th World Vet. Congress Hanover, Germany, *2*:1117, 1963.
21. Henry, W. B., Sieber, S. E.: Traumatic diabetes insipidus in a dog. J. Am. Vet. Med. Assoc., *146*:1317, 1965.
22. Ivy, H. K.: The syndrome of inappropriate secretion of antidiuretic hormone. Med. Clin. North Am., *52*:817, 1968.
23. Koestner, A., and Capen, C. C.: Ultrastructural evaluation of the canine hypothalamic-neurohypophysial system in diabetes insipidus associated with pituitary neoplasms. Pathol. Vet., *4*:513, 1967.
24. Lauson, H. D., Bocanegra, M., and Beuzeville, C. F.: Hepatic and renal clearance of vasopressin from plasma of dogs. Am. J. Physiol., *209*:199, 1965.
25. Lloyd, S., and Pickford, M.: The vascular responses to neurohypophyseal hormones of rats and dogs with abnormal sexual development. J. Physiol., *168*:932, 1963.
26. Miller, M., and Moses, A. M.: Mechanism of chlorpropamide action in diabetes insipidus. J. Clin. Endocrinol. Metab., *30*:488, 1970.
27. Mills, E., and Wang, S. C.: Liberation of antidiuretic hormone: location of ascending pathways. Am. J. Physiol., *207*:1399, 1964.
28. Moses, A. M.: Synthetic lysine vasopressin nasal spray in the treatment of diabetes insipidus. Clin. Pharmacol. Ther., *5*:422, 1964.
29. Moses, A. M., and Miller, M.: Urine and plasma osmolality in diagnosis and management of dilutional hyponatremia. Postgrad. Med., *52*:232, 1972.
30. Murase, T., and Yoshida, S.: Mechanism of chlorpropamide action in patients with diabetes insipidus. J. Clin. Endocrinol. Metab., *36*:174, 1973.
31. Navar, L. G., Uther, J. B., and Baer, P. G.: Pressure diuresis in dogs with diabetes insipidus. Nephron, *8*:97, 1971.
32. Nawar, T., and Genest, J.: Non-hormonal drugs for the treatment of diabetes insipidus. Can. Med. Assoc. J., *107*:1225, 1972.

33. Potter, W. R.: Diabetes insipidus in the dog. Vet. Rec., *76*:438, 1964.
34. Rallison, M. L., and Tyler, F. H.: Treatment of diabetes insipidus in children with lysine-8-vasopressin. J. Pediatr., *70*:122, 1967.
35. Relkin, R.: Diabetes insipidus. N. Y. State J. Med., *66*:2789, 1966.
36. Rosenbloom, A. L.: Chlorpropamide in diabetes insipidus in childhood. Curr. Ther. Res., *13*:671, 1971.
37. Ryden, G., and Sjoholm, I.: Half-life of oxytocin in blood of pregnant and non-pregnant women. Acta Endocrinol., *61*:425, 1969.
38. Saito, T., and Yoshida, S.: Levels of antidiuretic hormone in plasma after hemorrhage and infusion of hypertonic saline in dogs. Endocrinology, *88*:1511, 1971.
39. Sawin, C. T.: The Hormones. Little, Brown, and Company, Inc., Boston, 1969.
40. Sawyer, W. H., Chan, W. Y., and Van Dyke, H. B.: Antidiuretic responses to neurohypophysial hormones and some of their synthetic analogues in dogs and rats. Endocrinology, *71*:536, 1962.
41. Schrier, R. W., et al.: Effect of isotonic saline infusion and acute haemorrhage on plasma oxytocin and vasopressin concentrations in dogs. Clin. Sci., *35*:433, 1968.
42. Share, L., and Levy, M. N.: Cardiovascular receptors and blood titer of antidiuretic hormone. Am. J. Physiol., *203*:425, 1962.
43. Shu'Ayb, W. A., Moran, W. H., and Zimmermann, B.: Studies of the mechanism of antidiuretic hormone secretion and the post-commissurotomy dilutional syndrome. Ann. Surg., *162*:690, 1965.
44. Spellacy, W. N., et al.: Growth hormone release in response to injected oxytocin or insulin. Obstet. Gynecol., *36*:82, 1970.
45. Taclob, L. T., and Needle, M. A.: Hyponatremic syndromes. Med. Clin. North Am., *57*:1425, 1973.
46. Thorn, N. A., and Smith, M. W.: Renal excretion of synthetic arginine-vasopressin injected into dogs. Acta Endocrinol., *49*:388, 1965.
47. Usami, S., Peric, B., and Chien, S.: Release of antidiuretic hormone due to common carotid occlusion and its relation with vagus nerve. Proc. Soc. Exp. Biol. Med., *111*:189, 1962.
48. Webster, B., and Bain, J.: Antidiuretic effect and complications of chlorpropamide therapy in diabetes insipidus. J. Clin. Endocrinol. Metab., *30*:215, 1970.
49. Wiederman, J., Freund, M., and Stone, M. L.: Oxytocin effect on myoepithelium of the breast throughout pregnancy. J. Appl. Physiol., *19*:310, 1964.
50. Wiggelinkhuizen, J., et al.: Nephrogenic diabetes insipidus and obstructive uropathy. Am. J. Dis. Child., *126*:398, 1973.
51. Yoshida, S., Ibayashi, H., Murakawa, S., and Nakao, K.: Cerebral control of secretion of antidiuretic hormone: effect of electrical stimulation of the prepyriform area on the neurohypophysis in the dog. Endocrinology, *77*:597, 1965.
52. Yoshida, S., Ibayashi, H., Murakawa, S., and Nakao, K.: Cerebral control of antidiuretic hormone release: effect of electrical stimulation of the medial aspect of the dog brain. Endocrinology, *79*:871, 1966.

Chapter 7

The Thyroid Gland

The thyroid gland is composed histologically of two important cellular configurations. The *follicle,* the predominant structure in the thyroid gland, is a single row of columnar epithelial cells surrounding homogeneous staining colloid. It is the functional unit that produces and secretes the classic thyroid hormones involved in calorigenic activity. The colloid contains thyroglobulin, a peptide that is a storage form of the thyroid hormones. Other important histologic cells in the thyroid gland are the *parafollicular* or C cells, which secrete calcitonin.

ANATOMY

The canine thyroid gland consists of two separate lobes, which lie laterally and slightly ventrally on the trachea. In the rare exception there is an isthmus connecting them. The lobes lie over the third to eighth tracheal rings, and they are flattened dorsolaterally. Unless the thyroid is enlarged, it is not palpable.

In addition to the two major lobes of the canine thyroid, aberrant thyroid tissue may be present. This tissue may lie anterior to the thyroid, and be incorporated within the remnants of the thyroglossal duct, or it may lie posterior to the thyroid along the trachea, following it into the thorax. Aberrant thyroid tissue has also been known to exist within the pericardium.

PHYSIOLOGY

The control of thyroid function appears to be mainly a function of the hypothalamus, which is sensitive to changing levels of free thyroid hormones. Decreasing levels of circulating free thyroid hormones stimulate secretion of thyrotropin-releasing factor (TRF) in the hypothalamus. TRF is carried via the hypothalamo-adenohypophyseal portal system to the anterior pituitary gland where it stimulates the synthesis and release of thyrotropin (TSH). The latter is transported in the blood to the thyroid gland, where it stimulates the biosynthesis and secretion of thyroid hormones.

The major function of the thyroid gland is the production, storage, and release of hormones that are intimately involved in the normal metabolic processes of cells in general. The thyroid responds readily to increased demands for its hormone production, and maintains a constant production of these hormones despite a wide variation in iodine intake. From the standpoint of function, the thyroid can be described as an organ that concentrates inorganic iodine from the blood, oxidizes and incorporates the iodine into thyroid hormone, and temporarily stores the hormones in the thyroid follicle. Eventually the hormones are released into the circulation. In man there are two major hormones, thyroxine (T_4) and triiodothyronine (T_3). Although circulating levels of T_3 are present in the dog, the physiologic significance of this hormone has not been determined.

Thyrotropin-Releasing Factor

Recent identification of the hypothalamic origin of TRF and the elucidation of its chemical structure have greatly expanded the understanding of thyroid physiology. TRF is a small peptide with a relatively simple structure, and it has been synthesized. Although TRF stimulates TSH secretion, the specificity is still unclear. Some evidence suggests that TRF administration does not affect the secretion of FSH and LH, whereas other reports have indicated that a significant increase in LH concentration in the serum occurs following infusion of TRF. The increased secretion of LH was small but significant. Since the synthesis of TRF is a relatively recent development, its actions have not been completely delineated.

Thyrotropin (TSH)

Thyrotropin, a peptide, is measurable by means of radioimmunoassay procedures. However, most TSH radioimmunoassay procedures are based on the immunologic response to purified human TSH. The structure of canine TSH has not been determined, and its similarities and dissimilarities to human TSH are not known. In the future, if canine TSH becomes available, it will be possible to determine whether there is cross immunologic activity between canine and human TSH. Until this matter is clarified, caution should be exercised in determining TSH levels in the dog by means of assay procedures that utilize human TSH as the standard material.

Hormonal Biosynthesis and Release

Inorganic iodine is absorbed from the gastrointestinal tract into the blood. Together with iodide obtained from the breakdown of thyroid hormone, it provides a source of serum iodide. The thyroid selectively extracts iodide, and excessive amounts are excreted by the kidney. Iodide is oxidized to iodine in the epithelial cells of the thyroid, and it immediately combines with tyrosine to form monoiodotyrosine and diiodotyrosine. Subsequently, two molecules of diiodotyrosine combine to form one molecule of thyroxine (T_4). The latter is secreted into the blood, or combines with a peptide to form thyroglobulin, which is stored within the colloid. Combination of monoiodotyrosine and diiodotyrosine results in the formation of triiodothyronine (T_3), which is also stored in thyroglobulin.

T_4 and T_3 are released from stored thyroglobulin by a hydrolytic enzyme, a protease, which disrupts their combination with thyroglobulin and thus permits their passage into the blood where they combine with plasma proteins. Thyroglobulin is rarely found in the blood except in certain pathologic processes in which the thyroid has been damaged. The presence of T_3 in the canine circulation does not necessarily indicate that this substance is an active and physiologic compound. Its presence may also result from the deiodination of T_4, so it may be an inactive catabolite. In man, T_3 is approximately 2½ times more potent than T_4, and the ratio of T_4 to T_3 in serum is approximately three to one.

TSH stimulates both the uptake of iodide by the thyroid gland and the oxidation of iodide into molecular iodine. It also stimulates the incorporation of iodine into the active hormones, the proteolysis of thyroglobulin, and the release of thyroxine into the circulation.

Hormonal Transport

Thyroxine-binding proteins are physiologically important. Essentially, in man two major proteins have a high affinity for T_4, thyroxine-binding globulin (TBG) and thyroxine-binding prealbumin. Normally only a very small fraction (less than 0.1%) of T_4 in plasma is in the free state. The rate at which T_4 leaves plasma to enter tissues correlates with the free T_4 fraction, and is in turn inversely related to the T_4 binding capacity of plasma proteins. Thyroxine-binding proteins carry approximately 99.9% of the circulating thyroid hormones.

Detailed analysis of canine thyroxine-binding proteins have not been carried out. One study did show that, in canine serum, T_4 was bound to alpha-globulin, albumin, and material that moved electrophoretically just ahead of the beta-globulins. When the buffer system was changed, T_4 was bound only to albumin and alpha-globulin. In another study, T_4 was bound to three post-albumin zones in addition to albumin. Thyroxine-binding globulin or TBG-like protein is present in canine serum; however, its concentration is lower than that in other species.

All of the studies of thyroxine-binding proteins in the dog indicate that the binding capacity is not identical to that in man. Binding proteins transport sufficient levels of T_4 throughout the body where dissociation allows a continuous supply of free hormones for cellular metabolism.

Peripheral Hormone Metabolism

Thyroxine is carried to the tissues, and deiodinated at the cellular surface, the excess iodine returning to the blood where it is available for further hormone synthesis. The deiodination of T_4 results in the formation of T_3; in man this active compound becomes incorporated within the cell, increasing cellular metabolism. It is not known whether deiodination is necessary to produce this metabolic effect since both T_4 and T_3 have biologic activity, the latter a much greater and more rapid action. The metabolites of T_4 and T_3 are conjugated by the liver and excreted with bile into the intestinal tract where they are reabsorbed and reutilized.

Normal metabolic homeostasis results from a balance between the rate of hormone production and its release by the thyroid, the latter being mediated through the release of TSH by the pituitary gland. There is no general agreement as to the relative importance of the tissues, the thyroid, or the pituitary in this cycle. Regardless of the primary stimulus to thyroid gland secretion, there is a close reciprocal relationship between the thyroid and the pituitary; e.g., increased TSH production causes hyperplasia of the thyroid, and decreased production causes involution. Similarly, the administration of T_4 to a euthyroid individual will reduce TSH production, whereas thyroidectomy causes increased TSH secretion by the pituitary.

LABORATORY TESTS

There are many assay procedures used in the study of thyroid physiology. Since this field is expanding rapidly, tests available in the near future will supplement or replace some of the tests described. Based on the present understanding of thyroid physiology, an important factor is the absolute free thyroxine level in serum. Since this fraction is considered important at the cellular level, a test for free serum thyroxine would be valuable.

Protein-Bound Iodine (PBI)

This test, which was one of the first and classic in vitro tests for thyroid function, chemically determines the amount of iodine that is co-precipitable with serum proteins. The reliability of the test is based on the assumption that the PBI value represented predominately hormonal iodine. However, various substances can interfere with PBI determinations and cause falsely high or low results.

Essentially all spuriously high PBI measurements are due to the presence of exogenous iodine, which is measured along with the PBI. Most radiographic dyes are organic iodine compounds; thus, they provide a frequent source of error. The duration of interference is about one week for dyes used in angiography and intravenous pyelography, and up to several months for some of the oil-based dyes used in myelography. Topical and oral preparations containing iodine are another source of error. The mercury content of some diuretics can cause an artificial decrease in the PBI level by interfering with the chemical assay of PBI.

Nonhormonal iodoproteins may be released into the circulation. Since a dog's nonhormonal iodoproteins appear to be quite abundant under some conditions, the PBI value is falsely elevated at those times. Because of the indirect nature of this test and the frequent false readings, a PBI test is not considered a reliable parameter of thyroid function.

Butanol Extractable Iodine (BEI)

The butanol extractable iodine test is slightly more specific than the PBI in that butanol extraction separates inorganic iodine and iodoproteins from T_4. This differential extraction increases the sensitivity and specificity of the method. However, radiographic dyes still cause interference. Although this test is superior in many ways to the PBI, it is an indirect method for the measurement of thyroxine. With the newer techniques that measure thyroxine levels directly, it is no longer used to any degree.

^{131}I Uptake

The radioactive iodine uptake test (RAI) uses a counting device to measure thyroid uptake of a tracer dose of an isotope of iodine, usually ^{131}I, given orally. Counting usually is carried out 24 and 48 hours after administration, at which times hypothyroidism and hyperthyroidism are most easily distinguished.

Although this test is useful in determining the functional ability of the thyroid to take up iodine, numerous factors have prevented it from becoming more widely used in veterinary medicine. One objection is that specialized equipment and strict precautions are required for handling radioactive isotopes, so the test has been restricted mainly to institutions. Moreover, it has recently been established that administration of radioactive iodine to animals and man increases the probability of thyroid carcinoma later in life.

The radioactive scan is often incorporated as part of an ^{131}I uptake determination, but need not be in all instances; ^{131}I, ^{123}I, and ^{99m}Tc(technetium) as sodium pertechnetate have been used for the radioisotope scan, and all give basically similar results. The scan is useful in diagnosis of masses in the neck, and also helps to visualize functioning aberrant thyroid tissue. An important use of the scanner is to determine whether a thyroid tumor is functional. In man, functional or "hot" nodules are almost never malignant. This statement is not true for dogs; their functional thyroid tumors are often malignant. When a thyroid tumor readily picks up ^{131}I, the tumor is amenable to radioactive iodine therapy.

Basal Metabolic Rate (BMR)

This test was used for many years, mainly when it was the only measurable index of thyroid function. While this test was popular in human medicine, it lacked acceptability in veterinary medicine because it required a cooperative patient—one that would not struggle, yet could tolerate the equipment necessary for the study. This test is no longer used to any degree in human medicine since the advent of newer and more sophisticated techniques of directly measuring the specific hormones involved.

The BMR measures total metabolic activity under basal conditions, rather than thyroid activity per se. Consequently, it is influenced not only by drugs used in the treatment of diseases of the thyroid, but also by other medications. Thus, exposure to cold, disease states causing fever, as well as cardiopulmonary and blood diseases produce high basal metabolic rates in the absence of disease of the thyroid. Pituitary and gonadal failure may erroneously suggest a low level of thyroid activity. However, when obvious sources of inaccuracy are excluded and multiple determinations are performed, the accuracy of the BMR is increased.

^{131}I-Triiodothyronine (T_3) Resin Sponge Uptake

The T_3 Resin Sponge Uptake determination refers generically to a group of tests that indirectly reflect the level of both serum thyroxine and the binding proteins by measuring unoccupied sites on the binding protein. Despite its name, unfortunately abbreviated even further to T_3 test, this procedure has nothing to do with actual T_3 serum levels. The T_3 Resin Sponge Uptake and the actual T_3 level in serum are entirely different tests.

The T_3 Resin Sponge Uptake test is performed by mixing radioactively labeled T_3 with the serum sample. An ion exchange resin embedded in a sponge is added, and the distribution of labeled T_3 between the resin and the serum proteins is measured. The fewer available binding sites on the protein, the more T_3 has been absorbed by the resin. Since the number of available binding sites is determined not only by the amount of binding protein, but also by the amount of endogenous T_4 occupying some of the sites, the test is sensitive to both factors. In hyperthyroidism, for example, most of the protein sites are occupied because of the elevated T_4 levels; accordingly, the resin uptake of T_3 is increased. An identical increase in the resin uptake could occur in a euthyroid dog that has decreased amounts of binding proteins.

Although most circulating thyroid hormones are bound to specific plasma proteins, the bound hormone is in equilibrium with a very small fraction of the physiologically active, free hormone. The degree of saturation of the binding protein varies with the thyrometabolic state. In hyperthyroidism, the excessive production of hormone pushes the equilibrium toward further saturation of the binding proteins. Conversely, in hypothyroidism, the low production of hormone leaves the binding protein relatively unsaturated. Therefore, an assessment of circulating thyroid hormones can be inferred by measuring the degree of saturation of the binding proteins. Although the T_3 Resin Sponge Uptake test is a measurement of the degree of unsaturation of thyroxine-binding proteins, this test is more accurate when combined with a direct method for quantitating thyroxine. T_3 Resin Sponge Uptake values are higher in dogs than in man. Most studies in the dog report normal values of 45 to 55%.

Total Serum Thyroxine

Recently many procedures for directly measuring total serum thyroxine have become available. A number of these tests can be used with canine sera though others require extensive modification to be accurate for quantitating T_4 in canine blood.

The *T_4 by column* technique removes interfering substances from T_4 chromatographically before the iodine content is measured. This procedure is an improvement over the PBI and BEI, but it is still subject to interference from some radiographic dyes. In addition, the routine laboratory procedure set up for human samples would need major modification to assess the low levels of T_4 in canine serum.

Competitive protein-binding procedure for T_4 (Murphy-Pattee test, or the T_4-by-displacement test) does not rely on the chemical analysis of iodine. Rather the total thyroxine content of the serum is measured directly by a competitive protein-binding procedure that depends on the specific binding of thyroxine by TBG (thyroxine-binding globulin). The results are expressed in terms of the amount of thyroxine present and are usually stated in micrograms per 100 ml of blood. In the dog the normal range is 2.0 to 3.5 μg/100 ml. This test is specific and eliminates the problem of interference. It is also reliable and accurate, especially when slightly modified to increase the final amount of thyroxine measured because of the low levels of T_4 in canine serum.

Recently methods have been developed to measure *total serum thyroxine (T_4) by radioimmunoassay.* Radioimmunoassay procedures are sensitive and precise. The only interfering substances are those with similar chemical structures and cross-immunologic properties. In general, radioimmunoassay procedures are accurate.

Free Thyroxine Index

Using the T_3 Resin Sponge Uptake in conjunction with the Total Serum Thyroxine determination lets one estimate the free thyroxine level (Free Thyroxine Index or T_7 value) by multiplying the T_3 Resin Sponge Uptake percentage by the Total Serum Thyroxine value. The excellent correlation between the Free Thyroxine Index and the absolute level of free thyroxine as measured by dialysis makes the Free Thyroxine Index a useful measurement of thyroid function.

Effective Thyroxine Ratio

Recently another test has been used in human medicine; like the Free Thyroxine Index, it is highly correlated with the absolute level of free thyroxine. Its additional advantage is that just one test is needed to get the same type of correlative results. With this test the concentration of thyroxine in test serum is determined in the presence of the test serum itself; then it is expressed as a fraction of the thyroxine concentration similarly determined in normal serum. The ratio obtained is called "effective thyroxine ratio," which correlates precisely with the thyroid state irrespective of the serum-binding protein concentrations. If this test is used for canine blood, the total serum thyroxine level determined should be compared to a normal canine serum sample.

Antithyroglobulin Autoantibodies

Thyroglobulin, the principal protein comprising the colloid, cannot escape from the follicle except when the epithelial walls are disrupted by disease. Being isolated from the rest of the body, thyroglobulin predictably stimulates autoantibody production in certain thyroid diseases, presumably due to disruption of the follicle. In a number of thyroid diseases in man, agglutinating autoantibodies to thyroglobulin have been demonstrated, as well as fluorescent autoantibodies, precipitins, and complement-fixing antibodies to various portions of thyroid epithelium. The presence of antibodies to either thyroglobulin or to thyroid epithelium has been well described in human medicine, but not in the veterinary medical literature.

Thyrotropin (TSH) Stimulation Test

Clinical application of TSH stimulation tests is based on the measurement of physiologic alterations caused by this hormone. Intramuscular administration of TSH increases both avidity of the normal thyroid gland for iodine and discharge of hormones from the gland. The latter can be measured directly.

The test can be used to differentiate the euthyroid dog from one with hypothyroidism. In the euthyroid animal a maximal response to TSH is usually seen 8 to 12 hours after administration. A response, though not maximal, is still present 24 hours postinjection. In a 24-hour response test 10 IU of diagnostic grade TSH are administered intramuscularly. Blood samples are taken prior to and 24 hours following injection. In the euthyroid animal the Total Serum Thyroxine increases in excess of 1.0 $\mu g\%$ over that of the preinjection level; usually the response is greater (mean increase = 3.1 ± 0.5 $\mu g\%$).

In most cases a single-dose TSH response test is sufficient to differentiate euthyroidism from hypothyroidism. An adequate response is seen in the normal animal, whereas in the hypothyroid dog this increase is minimal or absent. However, a less than normal increase does not differentiate pituitary or secondary hypothyroidism from primary hypothyroidism. To distinguish the two types, TSH must be administered for a longer period; three days is sufficient. With primary hypothyroidism, in which the defect lies within the thyroid gland itself, repeated administration of TSH does not produce an increased secretion of T_4. However, if hypothyroidism is caused by an insufficiency of endogenous TSH, although a single dose of exogenous TSH does not usually stimulate thyroxine secretion, repeated doses of TSH over three days usually produce a vigorous response.

Direct Measurement of Serum TSH

Serum level of TSH can be measured by radioimmunoassay. However, the available commercial tests for TSH use an antibody prepared against human TSH. It is not known whether canine TSH is immunologically similar to human TSH. When purified canine TSH becomes available, a specific assay for it could easily be established.

Direct Measurement of T_3

Although radioimmunoassay of serum triiodothyronine (T_3) is available, the physiologic significance of T_3 in the dog is not known; thus, any values obtained are of uncertain usefulness.

PATHOGENESIS OF HYPOTHYROIDISM

Hypothyroidism is the result of inadequate circulating thyroid hormones. It may be produced by a number of different biochemical mechanisms that may or may not be related to certain pathologic changes. Some causes of hypothyroidism are thyroid agenesis (athyroidism), enzymatic dyshormonogenesis or defects in biosynthesis, defects in tissue response to thyroid hormones, and destructive diseases of the thyroid gland, such as thyroiditis or neoplasia.

The thyroid hormones play a dominant role in controlling metabolism, and are essential for normal growth and development. Clinical features and laboratory findings indicative of hypothyroidism appear when the amounts of these hormones available to tissues and cells are insufficient.

The term dyshormonogenesis implies a disturbance of normal hormone production. While it may be due to a lack of stimulating action of TSH, as in pituitary hypothyroidism, or to insufficiency of dietary iodine, as in endemic hypothyroidism, it is especially due to a defect in the intrathyroidal mechanisms, in particular an abnormality in thyroid hormone synthesis. Theoretically, hypothyroidism may also result from a defect in the mechanism transporting thyroid hormones from the thyroid gland to the peripheral tissues, and from a defect in tissue cells which render them incapable of responding to normal levels of thyroid hormones in the blood.

Athyreosis

Hypothyroidism developing in utero, or during the early months following birth, severely affects the central nervous tissue. In addition, physical stunting results from the insufficiency of thyroid hormones. Thyroid agenesis or athyroidism results from a congenital defect in the development of the thyroid gland; in this condition, the gland is either completely absent or is so poorly developed that only remnants are present. Congenital hypothyroidism in man is called cretinism. Although described in the dog, its rarity suggests that affected puppies almost never survive. Severe lethargy and unthriftiness of the affected pup often lead to early death from either secondary complications or euthanasia.

Thyroid agenesis is distinguished pathologically from enzymatic dyshormonogenesis by the larger thyroid gland in the latter. The decreased feedback of the thyroid hormones stimulates an increased secretion of TSH, which produces hyperplasia and enlargement of the thyroid gland. With thyroid agenesis, the thyroid gland is not palpable.

Dyshormonogenesis

Defects in the biosynthesis of hormones due to insufficiency of specific enzymes are well described in human medicine. Many of these disorders are inherited. Numerous types of intrathyroidal defects have been differentiated, for example, (1) a defect in the thyroid gland's mechanism for trapping iodine; (2) defective oxidation to and utilization of iodine to form monoiodotyrosine and diiodotyrosine; (3) defective coupling of monoiodotyrosine and diiodotyrosine with a resulting defect in the production of thyroxine or triiodothyronine; (4) defective production of thyroglobulin with the formation of an abnormal iodinated protein; and (5) defective proteolysis of thyroglobulin, which keeps stored thyroglobulin from being broken down to release thyroxine into the circulation. All dyshormonogenetic defects result in an inability to produce sufficient levels of active circulating thyroid hormones. These disorders, although seen in man, have not been described in the dog.

Defects in Transport of Thyroid Hormones

The thyroid hormones are carried in the peripheral blood bound to plasma proteins. Man has a specific thyroxine-binding globulin, which has a high affinity for thyroxine. Although evidence suggests that the binding of thyroxine in serum is not as strong in the dog as in man, it appears that protein binding of thyroid hormones in the dog is an important physiologic function.

Abnormalities in thyroxine-binding proteins have been described in man. Results of laboratory tests that I have performed in the clinic suggest that abnormalities in transport of the thyroid hormones also exist in the dog. However, alterations in thyroxine-binding proteins by themselves should not cause a clinical abnormality. With increasing levels of thyroxine-binding proteins and a normal pituitary-thyroid axis, the resulting decrease in circulating free thyroid hormones stimulates an increased secretion of TRF and TSH, followed by an increased secretion of thyroid hormones until free levels are re-established in the physiologic range.

A common finding in dogs with clinical signs of hypothyroidism is normal total serum thyroxine levels and decreased T_3 Resin Sponge Uptakes. These data suggest an increase in unsaturated binding sites on the thyroxine-binding proteins, and a decrease in free thyroxine in the circulation. These dogs respond dramatically to the administration of exogenous thyroxine. A possible explanation is that these animals have an increase in the thyroxine-binding proteins and *no* compensatory increase in total serum thyroxine which produces a normal free thyroxine level. This type of hypothyroidism is common in the dog, but the specific mechanism and the precise characteristics of the defect need further investigation.

Thyroiditis

Varying degrees of canine thyroiditis have been found on routine necropsy in animals that did not show signs of thyroid dysfunction. Chronic lymphocytic thyroiditis closely resembling Hashimoto's

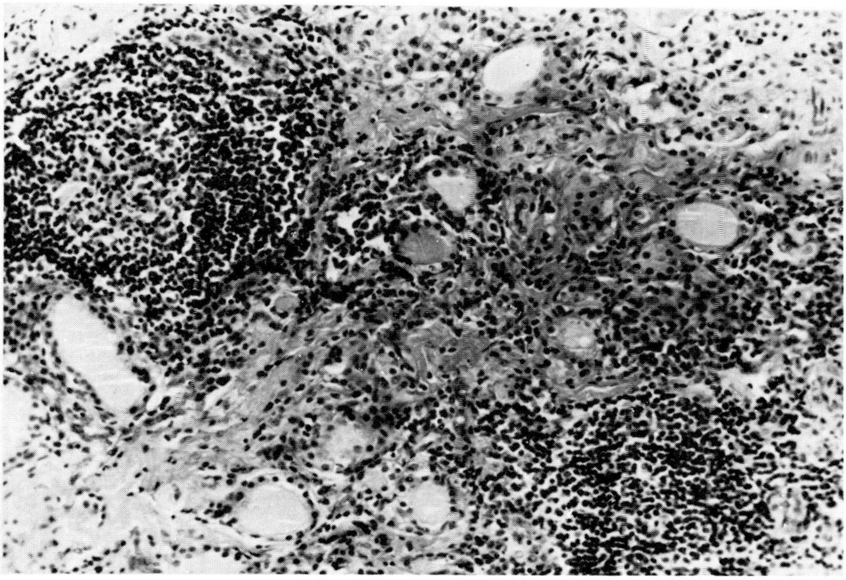

Fig. 7–1. Lymphocytic thyroiditis ×102. Follicular atrophy and infiltration with mononuclear cells, predominately lymphocytes. (Courtesy John T. McGrath, University of Pennsylvania.)

thyroiditis of man has also been described in the dog (Fig. 7–1). This type of thyroiditis is believed to be an autoimmune disease.

The clinical signs of chronic thyroiditis may be insidious in onset or may be imperceptible until alterations in the thyroid become quite extensive. In Hashimoto's thyroiditis the thyroid may become diffusely involved and moderately enlarged due to hyperplasia and lymphoid infiltration. In another type of human thyroiditis, called Reidel's struma, marked fibrosis and cellular destruction result in a thyroid gland that is smaller than normal and usually quite hard. Although thyroiditis is seen in the dog, its significance in the pathogenesis of the thyroid dysfunction is not clear.

Neoplasms

The main types of thyroid neoplasm are the follicular and medullary tumors. The papillary tumor has not been a consistent finding in the dog. Medullary carcinoma is quite different from other thyroid cancers. In man it is a solid tumor composed of islands of regular cells with an abundant granular cytoplasm and a variable amount of amyloid in the stroma. This type of tumor is derived from parafollicular cells, which normally secrete calcitonin. Medullary carcinoma in man has been shown to be capable of producing hypercalcitoninemia. These tumors may also be associated with multiple neural tumors and bilateral pheochromocytomas. Medullary carcinoma in man is familial and can secrete histaminase, prostaglandins, and serotonin, in addition to calcitonin.

Although the histologic appearance of predominately solid and well-differentiated thyroid tumors in the dog resembles medullary carcinoma of man, the lesion in the dog does not contain amyloid. Some investigators have tried to avoid the diagnosis of medullary carcinoma for this reason, and instead have classified these as a more noncommittal, "solid canine thyroid tumor" (Fig. 7–2). The functional activity of these tumors in the dog has not been studied to date.

All reported instances of thyrotoxicosis in the dog have been associated with thyroid tumors (Fig. 7–3). Clinical signs result from the hypersecretion of thyroid hormones by the autonomous tumors. Many hyperfunctional thyroid tumors in the dog are malignant. In man thyrotoxicosis is rarely caused by thyroid carcinoma.

When feasible, surgical treatment of thyroid tumors is preferred. However, when a thyroid tumor is hyperfunctional and the tumor will take up iodine, therapy with radioactive iodine (^{131}I) is theoretically possible. Only tumors that take up iodine respond to this type of therapy, and they usually are the follicular type.

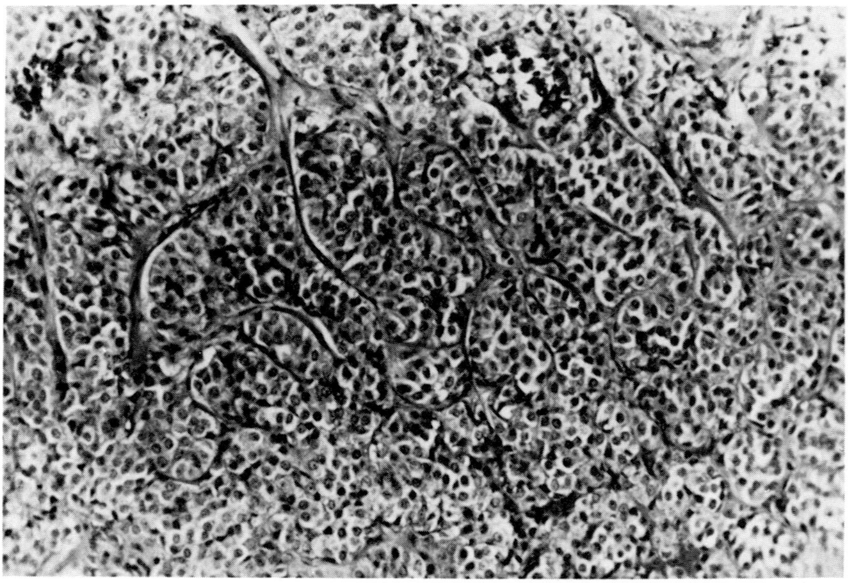

Fig. 7–2. "Solid-type" thyroid adenoma ×102. Islands of neoplastic epithelial elements are present without any follicular formation. (Courtesy John T. McGrath, University of Pennsylvania.)

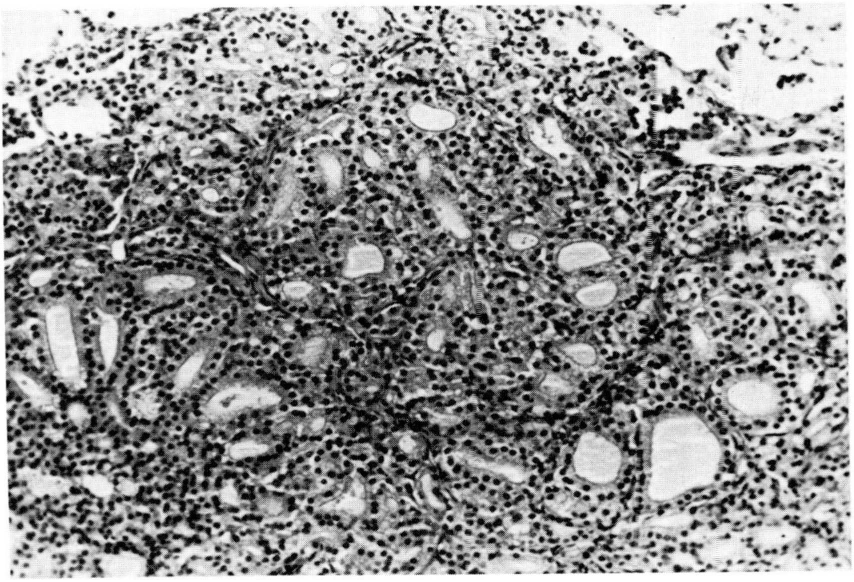

Fig. 7–3. Thyroid adenocarcinoma ×102. This tumor contains typical follicular formation. (Courtesy John T. McGrath, University of Pennsylvania.)

Deficient Production of TSH

When secretion of TSH is inadequate, the mechanism of trapping iodine for synthesizing thyroid hormones becomes defective. A deficiency of TSH is often accompanied by deficiencies of other anterior pituitary factors, i.e., ACTH, growth hormone, and gonadotropins. Occasionally there is an isolated deficiency of TSH, producing secondary hypothyroidism. This form of hypothyroidism can be distinguished from primary hypothyroidism by the affected animal's response to administration of exogenous TSH. In hypothyroidism resulting from an insufficiency of TSH, the thyroid gland, although possibly atrophied, remains responsive to a three-day TSH stimulatory test. In contrast, a response to TSH does not occur with primary hypothyroidism, regardless of the amount of TSH administered.

Peripheral Defects

It is difficult to prove the existence of a peripheral defect in the action of thyroid hormones in cases of hypothyroidism. Theoretically, peripheral defects may result from such mechanisms as failure of the hormones to cross the cell membrane to the site of action within the cell, or from actual failure of the peripheral tissue itself to respond to the thyroid hormones. The literature suggests that peripheral-defect hypothyroidism does occur in man, but there are no reported cases in the literature of veterinary medicine.

Decreased Absorption of Thyroxine

Among the many documented cases of hypothyroidism in the dog, a small percentage of these animals did not respond to the administration of exogenous *oral* sodium levothyroxine. Even after massive dosages of thyroxine, circulating levels of thyroxine did not increase. When thyroxine is given intramuscularly, the total serum thyroxine level and Free Thyroxine Index become elevated, suggesting a failure in absorption of thyroxine rather than an increased catabolism. Since parenteral administration of thyroxine is expensive, the prognosis is poor.

It is not known whether the primary defect in this type of hypothyroidism is the decreased intestinal absorption. Normally there is an enterohepatic circulation of thyroid hormones, and any abnormality resulting in a decreased absorption of thyroid hormones could lead to eventual hypothyroidism.

HYPOTHYROIDISM

Iodine Deficiency

Hypothyroidism is the result of inadequate circulating thyroid hormones. Since iodine is necessary for the formation of thyroid hormones, hypothyroidism may be caused by an absolute or relative deficiency in iodine intake or by treatment with drugs that prevent iodine utilization. Although iodine deficiency hypothyroidism has been described in certain localities, the widespread use of iodized salts in dog foods has made this type of disorder rare in most countries. The dog also appears to be somewhat protected against the development of iodine deficiency by its low renal clearance of iodine.

With iodine deficiency hypothyroidism, the decrease in circulating thyroid hormones stimulates a compensatory increased secretion of TSH. The latter results in a compensatory hyperplasia, producing an enlarged thyroid gland, a *goiter.* The term goiter signifies an enlargement of the thyroid gland without indicating the etiology. The enlargement may result from increased stimulation of the thyroid by TSH when levels of thyroid hormones in the serum are decreased, or it may result from inflammation caused by neoplastic invasion.

In iodine deficiency there is a low plasma level of inorganic iodine, an increased thyroid avidity for tracer doses of radioactive iodine, and a decreased secretion of thyroxine. Endemic goiter is the classic example of severe iodine deficiency. This type of hypothyroidism is seen in specific areas where iodine in the diet is below normal.

Primary Hypothyroidism

Primary hypothyroidism is an insufficiency in the secretion of the thyroid hormones resulting from disease in the thyroid gland itself. This dysfunction can be caused by athyroidism, by inherent metabolic defects of hormone formation, or by glandular destruction of the thyroid produced by inflammation, operation, or radiation. Primary hypothyroidism can be differentiated from secondary hypothyroidism by the response of the thyroid gland to exogenous TSH. Secondary hypothyroidism responds in three to five days after treatment with TSH, whereas primary hypothyroidism does not respond to TSH regardless of the length of time of administration.

Secondary (Pituitary) Hypothyroidism

Secondary hypothyroidism is caused by a pituitary dysfunction that reduces the stimulus for thyroid hormone formation. It is found associated with pituitary tumors and other diseases that destroy the pituitary. A deficiency of TSH in the adult dog is likely to be accompanied by evidence of deficiency of other anterior pituitary hormones. Secondary hypothyroidism is common in canine pituitary dwarfism.

Clinical Signs of Hypothyroidism

Clinical signs associated with hypothyroidism are the direct result of the hypometabolic state that develops from the insufficiency of the thyroid hormones in circulation. This insufficiency produces lethargy, intolerance to cold, changes in the skin and haircoat, abnormal estrous cycles, infertility, decreased libido, and gain in weight.

The most consistent clinical finding is lethargy; i.e., the animal sleeps most of each day or is reluctant to move. This lethargy is one of the first clinical signs to abate following replacement therapy. In fact, the animal becomes active within one to two weeks.

The intolerance to cold may be indicated if the animal seeks out warm locations within the house. In colder climates, affected dogs often are reluctant to go outside during the winter months and usually return to the warmth of the house as soon as possible. A decrease in body temperature is only occasionally seen in hypothyroid dogs.

If the haircoat is clipped, regrowth may take twice as long as usual. In some dogs the haircoat becomes thin and coarse, and the skin eventually feels thicker than normal (Fig. 7–4). However, the canine skin is not truly myxedematous, since the characteristic staining qualities of myxedema are not present. As the hair loss progresses, the alopecia may become somewhat bilaterally symmetrical, affecting primarily the trunk of the body. In some dogs hyperpigmentation of the skin may occur. As the skin becomes thickened, it may produce a puffy appearance around the eyes similar to that described in the

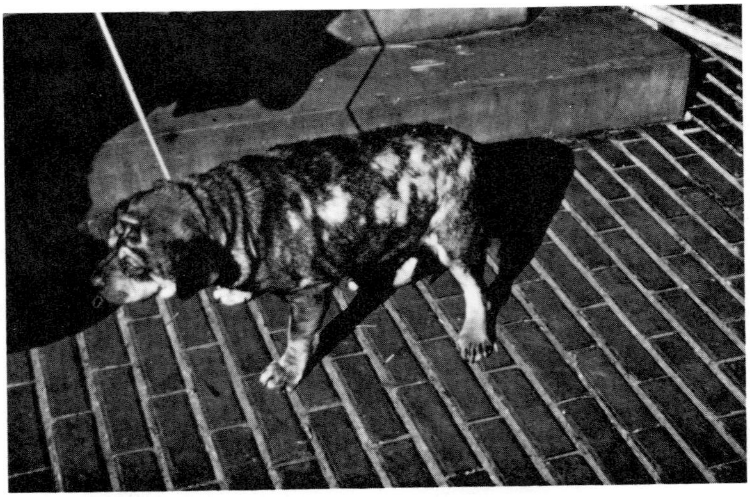

Fig. 7–4. Five-year-old mixed-breed dog with hypothyroidism. The haircoat is thin and coarse, affecting mainly the trunk of the body.

hypothyroid man, although this change over the face is not a consistent finding.

The estrous cycle is often affected in the intact hypothyroid bitch. Usually when the bitch comes into estrus, she does not attract as strongly as she would normally, and infertility is common. There is a decrease in libido in the male dog, and usually a decrease in the semen count.

Hypothyroid dogs are frequently normal in weight. However, if abnormal, the weight increase is associated with a normal or poorer than normal appetite (Fig. 7–5). In fact the absence of a ravenous appetite often is useful in differentiating hypothyroid obesity from exogenous obesity.

Decreased secretion of thyroid hormones results in decreased motility of the gastrointestinal tract and constipation. There have also been reports of cardiovascular changes with hypothyroidism in the dog, but they are unusual. In man there is usually a decrease in the heart rate and other electrocardiographic changes, such as decreased amplitude of all complexes and flattened or inverted T-wave.

TREATMENT OF HYPOTHYROIDISM

Preparations or extractions of animal thyroid glands were first used in the treatment of hypothyroidism in man over 70 years ago. Standard treatment for many years was the administration of desiccated thyroid, with the dosage being determined by the patient's clinical response

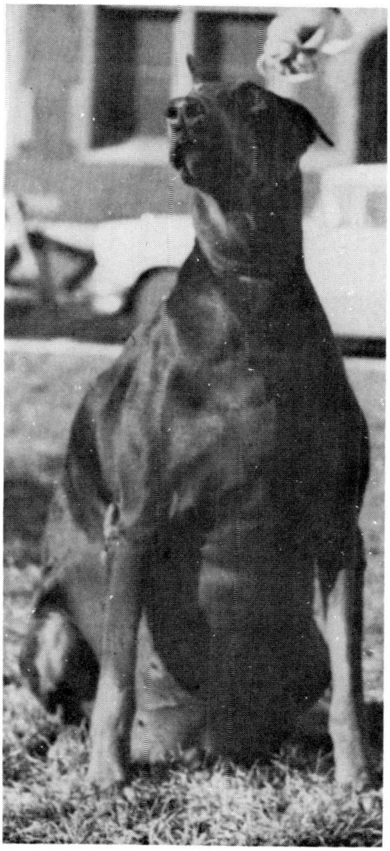

Fig. 7–5. Doberman pinscher (5½ years old, 172 pounds) with hypothyroidism. The dog consistently gained weight on a restrictive diet.

and his basal metabolic rate (BMR). In recent years, newer therapeutic agents have become available, and new test procedures have replaced the BMR evaluation.

There are essentially five major types of preparations used today in thyroid hormone replacement therapy: (1) desiccated thyroid preparations, (2) thyroglobulin, (3) sodium levothyroxine (T_4), (4) sodium liothyronine (T_3), and (5) a combination of T_3 and T_4 preparations. Desiccated thyroid medication is prepared from the thyroid glands of animals that have been slaughtered. This material contains 60 mg of desiccated thyroid preparation, standardized to contain from 20 to 30 μg of T_4 and 7 to 11 μg of T_3. One disadvantage of this preparation is its poor stability. Since its shelf-life is short, its usefulness is limited. Thyroglobulin has similar amounts of T_4 and T_3 and thus the similar instability of desiccated thyroid preparations.

Since sodium levothyroxine has been synthesized, it is widely used in treating hypothyroidism in the dog. It is relatively stable, and is active biologically in the dog. Usually 0.1 to 0.3 mg is administered twice daily per os. In small dogs (under 10 pounds), doses of 0.05 mg may be administered. Sodium levothyroxine must be given twice daily to maintain therapeutic blood levels.

Since the biologic activity of T_3 is in doubt in the dog, administration of sodium liothyronine (triiodothyronine, T_3) and/or the combination products containing T_4 and T_3 is questionable therapy. Some investigators have reported good results with the use of T_3 for replacement therapy, but others have not had the same experience.

Assessment of Free Thyroxine Index in the dog is useful in adjusting the replacement dosage in the hypothyroid patient. If a clinical response is not seen three to four weeks after an initial dose of the sodium levothyroxine, an additional determination of Free Thyroxine Index should be carried out while the animal is still on replacement therapy. In my experience, a clinical response is not usually observed if the Free Thyroxine Index is below normal. As the Free Thyroxine Index approaches the normal range, clinical signs abate. Following a satisfactory clinical response, the Free Thyroxine Index should be re-examined to prevent the possibility of an overdose. I recommend taking another blood sample two or three months after therapy is instituted.

PATHOGENESIS OF HYPERTHYROIDISM

Thyrotoxicosis is considered to be the second most common endocrine disease in man—diabetes mellitus being the first. The incidence of thyrotoxicosis in the dog is much lower. Although at one point the terms hyperthyroidism and thyrotoxicosis were used in slightly different ways, today they are used interchangeably. Hyperthyroidism is caused by excessive amounts of circulating thyroid hormones, and the toxic manifestations are related to increased metabolism.

Thyrotoxicosis has various causes; many human cases are associated with diffuse hyperplasia in which the specific etiology is still not well understood. Graves' disease in man is hyperthyroidism with an associated ophthalmopathy. Endocrine exophthalmos, the severe form of ocular proptosis with thyroid disease, occurs in only a small percentage of hyperthyroid cases. The hyperthyroidism of Graves' disease is maintained, if not initiated, by the interaction of an antibody (the long-acting thyroid stimulator (LATS)) and a thyroid antigen that is still uncharacterized. Thyrotropin appears to play no part in the establishment of Graves' disease; in fact, its secretion is suppressed in the normal physiologic way in this condition.

Little is known about the relationship between the effect of LATS and two major findings of Graves' disease, i.e., the ophthalmopathy and pretibial myxedema. The LATS most likely has a role, as yet undefined, in pretibial myxedema, but does not seem to have a direct pathogenic action in the ophthalmopathy. The mode of action of LATS on the thyroid is unknown. However, it does appear that LATS can activate the human thyroid. Therefore, it is reasonable to postulate that, once present in the blood, the stimulator is the cause of hyperthyroidism. One reason for controversy in understanding the pathogenesis of LATS in hyperthyroidism and/or Graves' disease is the few reported cases of exophthalmos without thyrotoxicosis. In these few, high levels of LATS were reported without the accompanying thyrotoxicosis.

TSH-Producing Pituitary Tumors

Thyrotoxicosis, secondary to a pituitary tumor secreting excessive amounts of TSH, is extremely rare. Reports on a few cases in man describe a chromophobe adenoma present in the pituitary. To my knowledge, no proven case of thyrotoxicosis in the dog has been established as due to excessive secretion of TSH by a pituitary tumor.

Triiodothyronine Thyrotoxicosis

As accurate methods have been developed for assaying T_3 in serum, the importance of this hormone in both normal and pathologic states has attracted considerable attention. The first report of T_3 hyperthyroidism in man was written in 1957; since then, this condition has been reported frequently. Clinical signs of thyrotoxicosis in the presence of a normal serum thyroxine level, and the absence of any abnormality of thyroxine-binding globulin, are suggestive of triiodothyronine hyperthyroidism. This type of thyrotoxicosis is treated similarly to other forms of hyperthyroidism. It is impossible to know whether T_3 thyrotoxicosis is a legitimate disorder in the dog. To date it has not been reported.

Functional Thyroid Tumors

All documented cases of thyrotoxicosis in the dog have been associated with autonomous functioning thyroid tumors. Diffuse thyroidal hyperplasia seen with Graves' disease in man has not been described with hyperthyroidism in the dog. Since thyrotoxicosis is often diagnosed in the dog only after finding an enlarged thyroid gland, it is possible that, with better methods of recognition, there will be reports of canine thyrotoxicosis without thyroid tumors. Biologically the functioning thyroid tumors in the dog are quite different from those in man. In the dog many hyperfunctional tumors are malignant, whereas in man they are usually benign. Tumors account for only 10% of the cases of thyrotoxicosis in man.

HYPERTHYROIDISM

Clinical Signs

The clinical findings of thyrotoxicosis are primarily those resulting from increased metabolism, e.g., weight loss (despite an increased appetite and food intake), varying degrees of heat intolerance, increased activity or excitability, weakness, diarrhea, polydipsia, and polyuria. The most consistent finding is severe weight loss. Polydipsia and polyuria are not present in all cases of canine thyrotoxicosis, but when present, they may be severe. The cause of the polyuria is due to the direct diuretic effect of thyroid hormones. Since hypercalcemia has been reported in a certain percentage of thyrotoxic individuals, and since hypercalcemia is known to cause polyuria, it may also contribute to the diuresis seen in some animals.

Diarrhea may be severe with hyperthyroidism since the thyroid hormones increase gastrointestinal tract motility. However, if hypercalcemia develops, constipation may result rather than diarrhea.

Cardiovascular changes are not consistently seen in canine thyrotoxicosis. Furthermore, experiments to produce cardiovascular changes in dogs by giving massive amounts of thyroxine have not been successful.

There have been no documented cases of exophthalmos associated with thyrotoxicosis in the dog. The few cases of exophthalmos reported did not involve pathologic changes in the eye similar to those reported in Graves' disease of man.

Thyroid Storm

Thyroid storm or thyroid crisis is generally defined as a sudden exaggeration of the manifestations of thyrotoxicosis; the symptoms actually reach life-threatening proportions. All the clinical signs are related to hypermetabolism. There may be uncontrollable hyperpyrexia; diarrhea; increased cardiac strain, which may lead to cardiac decompensation; progressive hepatic damage; and eventual coma. In man, the cardiovascular signs are quite prominent and usually include tachycardia, atrial fibrillation, premature ventricular contractions, congestive heart failure, and shock. There is usually prostration and extreme weakness. This condition is considered to be a life-threatening endocrine emergency and requires immediate therapy. If untreated, thyroid storm may lead to death. Cardiovascular changes are not usually seen with canine thyrotoxicosis, so these findings would not be expected even if thyroid storm should occur.

Although thyroid storm has not been described in the dog, there are many cases of uncontrollable hyperpyrexia of unknown etiology, so thyroid storm or crisis should be considered suspect.

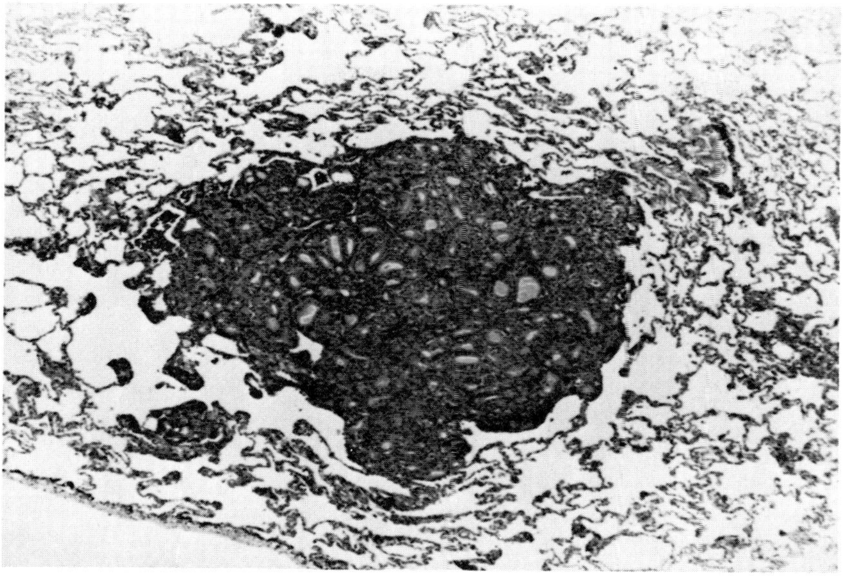

Fig. 7–6. Metastatic follicular thyroid adenocarcinoma in the lung (same dog as Fig. 7–3). Metastases were discovered on necropsy three years after removal of the primary thyroid tumor.

TREATMENT OF HYPERTHYROIDISM

Surgical Treatment

Since most thyrotoxic dogs have thyroid tumors, surgical removal is preferred, especially when the tumor is localized within the thyroid gland and can be removed completely. With tumors affecting only one lobe of the thyroid gland, surgical removal results in complete amelioration of clinical signs, and lifelong medication is not necessary. However, when tumors affect both lobes of the thyroid and are surgically removed, maintenance therapy is usually necessary for the life of the animal.

Thyroid tumors are rather slow-growing and they metastasize rather late (Fig. 7–6). If metastatic lesions are not present, surgical removal of the primary thyroid tumor is the treatment of choice.

Radioiodine Therapy

The use of high levels of ^{131}I for therapy of canine thyrotoxicosis will always be somewhat limited. The important factor in determining whether to administer radioiodine therapy is the presence of malignancy that actively concentrates the administered isotope. The tumor that picks up iodine is theoretically a candidate for radioisotopic therapy, but the inconvenience of using radioisotopes in animals hinders widespread application. Since those who use isotopes must be licensed, this type of therapy will probably gain acceptance in only a limited number of institutions.

One complication of ^{131}I therapy is the development of hypothyroidism after therapy. This condition is easily controllable by administration of exogenous thyroxine.

Antithyroid Drugs

Antithyroid drugs have gained wide acceptance in the therapy of benign thyrotoxicosis in man. Some of the advantages are that the patient does not need to enter a hospital or alter his daily routine following therapy. The antithyroid drugs also leave the thyroid gland intact, and most important, permanent complications are relatively rare.

There are essentially three common types of drugs used as antithyroid medications: the imidazole derivatives, thiouracil derivatives, and potassium perchlorate. The latter has been relatively abandoned in recent years because of the occasional occurrence of bone marrow depression.

When utilizing antithyroid drugs for inoperable thyrotoxicosis, it is judicious to begin with minimal doses, increasing as necessary to maintain euthyroidism. With present thyroid function studies, it is possible to monitor animals closely. As signs of thyrotoxicosis recur, the dosage of medication is increased accordingly.

Unfortunately, some antithyroid preparations have been used indiscriminately in veterinary medicine for diseases that have no well-documented association with thyroid hyperfunction. Propylthiouracil, a thiouracil derivative, has been reported effective in the treatment of acanthosis nigricans in the dog. Using potent antithyroid drugs for this disorder does not appear to be justified, and should be discouraged.

SELECTED READING

1. Abreau, C., et al.: A single method for measuring total thyroxine and free thyroxine index in serum. J. Nucl. Med., *14*:740, 1973.
2. Ahn, C. S., Athans, J. C., and Rosenberg, I. N.: Effects of epinephrine and of alteration in glandular blood flow upon thyroid function: studies using thyroid vein cannulation in dogs. Endocrinology, *84*:501, 1969.
3. Andersen, A. C., and Johnson, R. M.: Carcinoma of the thyroid in a beagle. Am. J. Vet. Res., *25*:861, 1964.
4. Anderson, J. J. B., and Dorner, J. L.: Total serum thyroxine in thyroidectomized beagles, using ^{125}I-labeled thyroxine, and comparison of T-3 and T-4 tests. J. Am. Vet. Med. Assoc., *159*:760, 1971.
5. Arosenius, K. E., Derblom, H., and Nylander, G.: Thiouracil treatment in pregnancy and lactation in the dog. Acta Endocrinol., *40*:430, 1962.
6. Ashkar, F. S., and Abelove, W. A.: Serum thyroxine as an index of thyroid function. Postgrad. Med., *56*:80, 1974.

7. Ashkar, F. S., and Bezjian, A. A.: Use of normalized serum thyroxine (T_4N). J.A.M.A., *221*:1483, 1972.
8. Bartuska, D.: Evolving concepts of the genetics of thyroid disease — a review. Am. J. Med. Sci., *266*:249, 1973.
9. Beierwaltes, W. H., and Nishiyama, R. H.: Dog thyroiditis: occurrence and similarity to Hashimoto's struma. Endocrinology, *83*:501, 1968.
10. Belshaw, B. E., and Becker, D. V.: Necrosis of follicular cells and discharge of thyroidal iodine induced by administering iodide to iodine-deficient dogs. J. Clin. Endocrinol. Metab., *36*:466, 1973.
11. Bogdanove, E. M.: Regulation of TSH secretion. Fed. Proc. *21*:623, 1962.
12. Brodey, R. S., and Kelly, D. F.: Thyroid neoplasms in the dog. Cancer, *22*:406, 1968.
13. Buergelt, C. D. Mixed thyroid tumors in two dogs. J. Am. Vet. Med. Assoc., *152*:1658, 1968.
14. Bullock, L.: Protein bound iodine determination as a diagnostic aid for canine hypothyroidism. J. Am. Vet. Med. Assoc., *156*:892, 1970.
15. Burke, G.: The thyrotrophin stimulation test. Ann. Intern. Med., *69*:1127, 1968.
16. Bush, B. M.: Thyroid function tests in a group of euthyroid dogs. Res. Vet. Sci., *13*:177, 1972.
17. Cassidy, C. E.: The treatment for hyperthyroidism. Med. Clin. North Am., *46*:1201, 1962.
18. Chopra, I. J., Solomon, D. H., and Ho, R. S.: Competitive ligand-binding assay for measurement of thyronine-binding globulin (TBG). J. Clin. Endocrinol. Metab., *35*:565, 1972.
19. Clark, F., and Horn, D. B.: Assessment of thyroid function by the combined use of the serum protein-bound iodine and resin uptake of ^{131}I-triiodothyronine. J. Clin. Endocrinol. Metab., *25*:39, 1965.
20. Coffin, D. L., and Munson, T. O.: Endocrine diseases of the dog associated with hair loss. J. Am. Vet. Med. Assoc., *123*:402, 1953.
21. Cunliffe, W. J., et al.: A calcitonin-secreting thyroid carcinoma. Lancet, *2*:63, 1968.
22. Davis, P. J., and Handwerger, B. S.: Thyroid hormone binding in dog plasma. Endocrinology, *93*:1445, 1973.
23. Denckla, W. D.: Minimal O_2 consumption as an index of thyroid status: standardization of method. Endocrinology, *93*:61, 1973.
24. DiScala, V. A., Lippe, R. D., and Segal, R. L.: A simple reliable method for producing hypothyroidism in the dog and thyroid function tests in normal and hypothyroid dog. Endocrinology, *88*:504, 1971.
25. Dobyns, B. M., et al.: Malignant and benign neoplasms of the thyroid in patients treated for hyperthyroidism: a report of the cooperative thyrotoxicosis therapy follow-up study. J. Clin. Endocrinol. Metab., *38*:976, 1974.
26. Donovan, E. F., nad Venzke, W. G.: Hypothyroidism in the dog Norden News, *43*:14, 1968.
27. Dumlao, J. S.: Thyroid storm. Postgrad. Med., *56*:57, 1974.
28. Dunn, R. T., and Foster, L. B.: Radioimmunoassay of thyroxine in unextracted serum, by a single-antibody technique. Clin. Chem., *19*:1063, 1973.
29. Ekins, R. P.: Radioimmunoassay, protein-binding assay and other saturation assay techniques. Practitioner, *207*:312, 1971
30. Elewaut, A., Degyter, M., Eeckhout, E , and Vermeulen, A.: Evaluation of a free thyroxine index. Ann. Endocrinol., *34*:84, 1973.
31. Evans, T. C., Beierwaltes, W. H., and Nishiyama, R. H.: Experimental canine Hashimoto's thyroiditis. Endocrinology, *84*:641, 1969.
32. Farer, L. S., Robbins, J., Blumberg, B. S., and Rall, J. E.: Thyroxine-serum protein complexes in various animals. Endocrinology, *70*:686, 1962.
33. Fisher, D. A.: Advances in the laboratory diagnosis of thyroid disease. Part I. J. Pediatr., *82*:1, 1973.
34. Fisher, D. A.: Advances in the laboratory diagnosis of thyroid disease. Part II. J. Pediatr., *82*:187, 1973.
35. Gershon, M. D., Belshaw, B. E., and Nunez, E. A.: Biochemical, histochemical and ultrastructural studies of thyroid serotonin, parafollicular and follicular cells during development in the dog. Am. J. Anat., *132*:5, 1971.

36. Gharib, H., and Wahner, H. W.: Triiodothyronine hyperthyroidism. Postgrad. Med., *54*:77, 1973.
37. Gillquist, J., Karlberg, B., Sjodahl, R., and Tegler, L.: Preoperative treatment of hyperthyroidism. Acta Chir. Scand., *140*:23, 1974.
38. Gordon, D. L., et al.: The serum calcium level and its significance in hyperthyroidism: a prospective study. Am. J. Med. Sci., *268*:31, 1974.
39. Goyings, L. S., Reineke, E. P., and Schirmer, R. G.: Clinical diagnosis and therapy of hypothyroidism in dogs. J. Am. Vet. Med. Assoc., *141*:341, 1962.
40. Green, W. L.: Guidelines for the treatment of myxedema. Med. Clin. North Am., *52*:431, 1968.
41. Greve, J. H., and Gaafar, S. M.: Radiotriiodothyronine for the evaluation of experimentally induced hypothyroidism in dogs. Am. J. Vet. Res., *25*:1191, 1964.
42. Guillemin, R.: The adenohypophysis and its hypothalamic control. Annu. Rev. Physiol., *29*:313, 1967.
43. Hall, R. J., and Nelson, W. P.: Thyroid heart disease. Postgrad. Med., *44*:127, 1968.
44. Hamilton, C. R., Adams, L. C., and Maloof, F.: Hyperthyroidism due to thyrotropin-producing pituitary chromophobe adenoma. N. Engl. J. Med., *283*:1077, 1970.
45. Harris, J. C., and Oliner, L.: Simultaneous resin uptake studies of labeled thyroxine and triiodothyronine in thyroid disease. J. Nucl. Med., *7*:259, 1966.
46. Hausmann, W.: Treatment of hyperthyroidism. Hormones, *3*:313, 1972.
47. Hightower, D., and Chester, D. K.: Letters to the editor. J. Am. Vet. Med. Assoc., *164*:5, 1974.
48. Hightower, D., Kyzar, J. R., Chester, D. K., and Wright, E. M.: Replacement therapy for induced hypothyroidism in dogs. J. Am. Vet. Med. Assoc., *163*:979, 1973.
49. Hollander, C. S., Thompson, R. H., Barrett, P. V. D., and Berlin, N. I.: Repair of the anemia and hyperlipidemia of the hypothyroid dog. Endocrinology, *81*:1007, 1967.
50. Ingbar, S. H., and Galton, V. A.: Thyroid. Annu. Rev. Physiol., *25*:361, 1963.
51. Isaacs, G. H., Athans, J. C., and Rosenberg, I. N.: Effects of thyrotropin upon thyroidal iodide; studies using thyroid venous cannulation and two radioiodine isotopes. J. Clin. Invest., *45*:758, 1966.
52. Ismail, A. A., et al.: Extravascular circulation of thyroid hormones. Am. J. Physiol., *213*:1391, 1967.
53. Kallfelz, F. A.: The triiodothyronine-^{131}I resin sponge uptake test as an indicator of thyroid function in dogs. J. Am. Vet. Med. Assoc., *152*:1647, 1968.
54. Kallfelz, F. A.: Comparison of the ^{125}T-3 and ^{125}T-4 tests in the diagnosis of thyroid gland function in the dog. J. Am. Vet. Med. Assoc., *154*:22, 1969.
55. Kallfelz, F. A.: Determination of total serum thyroxine in the dog by competitive protein binding of labeled thyroxine. Am. J. Vet. Res., *30*:929, 1969.
56. Kallfelz, F. A.: Observations on thyroid gland function in dogs: response to thyrotropin and thyroidectomy and determination of thyroxine secretion rate. Am. J. Vet. Res., *34*:535, 1973.
57. Kallfelz, F. A., and Erali, R. P.: Thyroid function tests in domesticated animals: free thyroxine index. Am. J. Vet. Res., *34*:1449, 1973.
58. Kelley, S. T., Oehme, F. W., Hoffman, S. B.: Evaluation of selected commercial thyroid function tests in dogs. Am. J. Vet. Res., *35*:733, 1974.
59. Kotani, M., et al.: Demonstration of thyroglobulin in dog lymph. Endocrinology, *82*:1047, 1968.
60. Kral, F.: Treatment of some acquired alopecic and acanthotic skin disorders in dogs. Small Anim. Clinician, *3*:427, 1963.
61. Lange, M. J.: Thyroid swellings. Practitioner, *212*:193, 1974.
62. Larsen, P. R.: Triiodothyronine: review of recent studies of its physiology and pathophysiology in man. Metabolism, *21*:1073, 1972.
63. Larsen, P. R., Dockalova, J., Sipula, D., and Wu, F. M.: Immunoassay of thyroxine in unextracted human serum. J. Clin. Endocrinol. Metab., *37*:177, 1973.
64. Lewis, R. M.: Models of auto-immunity. Postgrad. Med., *43*:143, 1968.
65. Lombardi, M. H., Comar, C. L., and Kirk, R. W.: Diagnosis of thyroid gland function in the dog. Am. J. Vet. Res., *23*:412, 1962.

66. Maenpaa, J.: Congenital hypothyroidism. Arch. Dis. Child., *47*:914, 1972.
67. Malamos, B., Miras, C. J., Karli-Samouilidou, J. N., and Koutras, D. A.: The serum tyrosine level as an index of thyroid function. J. Endocrinol., *35*:223, 1966.
68. Manning, P. J., Corwin, L. A., Jr., and Middleton, C. C.: Familial hyperlipoproteinemia and thyroid dysfunction of beagles. Exp. Mol. Pathol., *19*:378, 1973.
69. Matsuda, K., Shimoda, S. I., and Greer, M. A.: Demonstration of diiodotyrosine secretion from the dog thyroid gland. Life Sci., *3*:251, 1964.
70. McConahey, W. M.: Hashimoto's thyroiditis. Med. Clin. North Am., *56*:885, 1972.
71. Milhaud, G., Coutris, G., and Tubiana, M.: Le cancer medullaire de la thyroide et le syndrome d'hyperthyrocalcitonie. Presse Med., *77*:2129, 1969.
72. Nagataki, S., et al.: Triiodothyronine and thyroxine in thyroid glands of euthyroid Japanese subjects. J. Clin. Endocrinol. Metab., *35*:18, 1972.
73. Nauman, J., and Nauman, A.: The "effective thyroxine ratio" — new in vitro test of thyroid function and its correlation with free thyroxine. Acta Endocrinol., *76*:83, 1974.
74. Nishiyama, H., Sodd, V. J., Berke, R. A., and Saenger, E. L.: Evaluation of clinical value of ^{123}I and ^{131}I in thyroid disease. J. Nucl. Med., *15*:261, 1974.
75. Norris, W. P., Fritz, T. E., and Taylor, J. A.: Cycle of accommodation to restricted dietary iodide in the thyroid gland of the beagle dog. Am. J. Vet. Res., *31*:21, 1970.
76. Patel, Y. C., and Burger, H. G.: Serum triiodothyronine in health and disease. Clin. Endocrinol., *2*:339, 1973.
77. Pickrell, J. A., et al.: Evaluation of hypothyroidism in a beagle dog colony. Adv. Automated Analyses/Biomedical Profiling, *3*:143, 1970.
78. Quinlan, W., Jr., and Michaelson, S. M.: Iodine-131 uptake and protein-bound iodine in normal adult beagles. Am. J. Vet. Res., *28*:179, 1967.
79. Rabinowitz, J. L., Banks, W. C., and Greenberg, C. M.: Confirmation of a new, rapid, reliable test of thyroid function in dogs. Am. J. Vet. Res., *25*:1314, 1964.
80. Refetoff, S., Robin, N. I., and Fang, V. S.: Parameters of thyroid function in serum of 16 selected vertebrate species: a study of PBI, serum T_4, free T_4, and the pattern of T_4 and T_3 binding to serum proteins. Endocrinology, *86*:793, 1970.
81. Reid, C. F.: Thyroid function tests in the dog. J. Am. Vet. Med. Assoc., *155*:1571, 1969.
82. Riddell, P. E., and Robinson, G. A.: Thyroidal iodine-131 uptakes in purebred beagles and crossbred beagle-cairn terriers, with possible genetic mediation of uptake in the beagles. Am. J. Vet. Res., *26*:328, 1965.
83. Rijnberk, A.: Iodine metabolism and thyroid disease in the dog. Ph.D. Thesis, University of Utrecht, Utrecht, 1971.
84. Rijnberk, A., and der Kinderen, P. J.: Toxic thyroid carcinoma in the dog. Acta Endocrinol. [Suppl.] (Kbh.), *138*:177, 1969.
85. Rijnberk, A., and Van Der Horst, C. J. G : Investigations on iodine metabolism of normal and goitrous dogs. Zentralbl. Veterinaermed., *16*:495, 1969.
86. Robbins, J.: Radioassay and the thyroid gland. Metabolism, *22*:1021, 1973.
87. Roberts, K. E., et al.: Effect of phosphate in enhancing the action of triiodothyronine. Endocrinology, *59*:565, 1956.
88. Rocmans, P. A., Govaerts, M. J. M., and Dumont, J. E.: Metabolism of the dog's thyroid in vivo and in vitro. J. Endocrinol., *37*:345, 1967.
89. Schneider, P. B.: Laboratory examination of the thyroid. Postgrad. Med., *56*:91, 1974.
90. Schussler, G. C., and Plager, J. E.: Effect of preliminary purification of ^{131}I-thyroxine on the determination of free thyroxine in serum. J. Clin. Endocrinol. Metab., *27*:242, 1967.
91. Shively, J. N., and Epling, G. P.: Fine structure of the thyroid gland of young dogs. Am. J. Vet. Res., *30*:219, 1969.
92. Shively, J. N., Phemister, R. D., and Epling, G. P.: Fine structure of thyroid epithelium of young dogs treated with thyrotropin. Am. J. Vet. Res., *30*:229, 1969.
93. Siegel, E. T.: Letters to the editor. J. Am. Vet. Med. Assoc., *164*:5, 1974.
94. Siler, T. M., Yen, S. S. C., Vale, W., and Guillemin, R.: Inhibition by somatostatin on the release of TSH induced in man by thyrotropin-releasing factor. J. Clin. Endocrinol. Metab., *38*:742, 1974.

95. Singer, P. A., and Nicoloff, J. T.: Estimation of the triiodothyronine secretion rate in euthyroid man. J. Clin. Endocrinol. Metab., *35*:82, 1972.
96. Sparagana, M., Phillips, G., and Kucera, L.: Serum thyroxine by competitive protein binding analysis: clinical, statistical and comparative evaluation. J. Clin. Endocrinol. Metab., *29*:191, 1969.
97. Stein, R. B., and Price, L.: Evaluation of adjusted total thyroxine (free thyroxine index) as a measure of thyroid function. J. Clin. Endocrinol. Metab., *34*:225, 1972.
98. Takeda, Y.: Hormonal effects on distribution and excretion of iodide-I^{131} in the dog. Am. J. Physiol., *206*:1237, 1964.
99. Taurog, A., Porter, J. C., and Thio, D. T.: Nature of the ^{131}I-compounds released into the thyroid veins of rabbits, dogs and cats, before and after TSH administration. Endocrinology, *74*:902, 1964.
100. Theran, P., Thornton, G. W., and Belshaw, B. E.: Case records of the Angell Memorial Animal Hospital. J. Am. Vet. Med. Assoc., *148*:562, 1966.
101. Thomson, R. A. E., and Michaelson, S. M.: A source of false iodine-131 uptake and protein bound iodine values in dogs. Am. J. Vet. Res., *28*:1623, 1967.
102. Torjesen, P. A., Haug, E., and Sand, T.: Effect of thyrotrophin-releasing hormone and serum levels of pituitary hormones in men and women. Acta Endocrinol., *73*:455, 1973.
103. Tucker, W. E., Jr.: Thyroiditis in a group of laboratory dogs. Am. J. Clin. Pathol., *38*:70, 1962.
104. Turek, I. S., and Rocha, J.: Oral thyrotropin-releasing hormone (TRH) in depressive illness. J. Clin. Pharmacol., *14*:612, 1974.
105. Uller, R. P., Van Herle, A. J., and Chopra, I. J.: Comparison of alterations in circulating thyroglobulin, triiodothyronine and thyroxine in response to exogenous (bovine) and endogenous (human) thyrotropin. J. Clin. Endocrinol. Metab., *37*:741, 1973.
106. Waldmann, T. A., Weissman, S. M., and Levin, E. H.: Effect of thyroid administration on erythropoiesis in the dog. J. Lab. Clin. Med., *59*:926, 1962.
107. Wellby, M., and O'Halloran, M. W.: Measurement of the plasma free thyroxine level as a test of thyroid function. Br. Med. J., *2*:668, 1966.
108. Wellby, M. L., O'Halloran, M. W., and Marshall, J.: A comparison of effective thyroxine ratio, free thyroxine index and free thyroxine concentration in correcting for thyroxine-binding abnormalities in serum. Clin. Endocrinol., *3*:63, 1974.
109. Werner, S. C., and Nauman, J. A.: The thyroid. Annu. Rev. Physiol., *30*:213, 1968.
110. West, C. D., Chavre, V. J., and Wolfe, M.: A simple method for estimating serum thyroxine concentration in thyroid disease and iodine-treated patients. J. Clin. Endocrinol. Metab., *26*:986, 1966.
111. Wilson, W. B.: Laboratory aids in the diagnosis of thyroid disease. South. Med. J., *59*:848, 1966.
112. Wolfe, H. J., et al.: C-cell hyperplasia preceding medullary thyroid carcinoma. N. Engl. J. Med., *289*:437, 1973.

Chapter

8

The Parathyroid Gland

ANATOMY

The parathyroid glands are small, yellowish or reddish tan, flattened, oval bodies that lie within or in close proximity to the thyroid gland. There are typically four parathyroid glands, although ectopic or additional parathyroids have been well described. Location of the parathyroid glands may vary, but usually the cranial parathyroids lie on the upper pole of the canine thyroid gland. The cranial parathyroids are easily observed, and can be separated from the underlying thyroid tissue. The posterior parathyroid glands lie on the medial aspect of the thyroid between the middle and posterior third of the thyroid gland. The posterior glands are imbedded within the thyroid tissue and are not easily removed.

Embryologically the posterior parathyroids arise in association with the thymus; they are found within the thyroid tissue as described, or they may follow the thymus in its descent into the mediastinum. The posterior glands, therefore, may on occasion be located anywhere between the bifurcation of the common carotid arteries and the mediastinum.

Histologically the parathyroid glands consist of two major types of epithelial cells, the chief or principal cells and the oxyphil cells. The chief cells, which possess a clear cytoplasm, are thought to be the hormone-secreting cells. Oxyphil cells have a granular cytoplasm, and stain intensely with certain acid dyes. The canine parathyroid contains chief cells exclusively. A variant of the chief cell is the "water-clear" cell, which contains small, rounded nuclei and abundant cytoplasm.

PHYSIOLOGY

The parathyroid gland participates in the regulatory mechanism of calcium and phosphorus metabolism. The hormone secreted by the parathyroid gland is parathormone (PTH), which elevates serum calcium concentration and increases excretion of phosphate by the kidney. PTH activity on calcium homeostasis is interrelated with the action of calcitonin (CT) and vitamin D.

Parathyroid Hormone (PTH)

PTH plays a major role in calcium homeostasis by maintaining the concentration of ionized calcium in the extracellular fluid at a constant level. It prevents any wide fluctuation of calcium levels by immediately correcting any fall in plasma calcium. In addition, PTH plays an important role in bone metabolism, specifically bone resorption. Parathyroidectomy produces a fall in the plasma calcium level and an increase in the plasma phosphate concentration. Conversely, administration of PTH produces hypercalcemia and hypophosphatemia.

The chemical structure of human, bovine, and porcine PTH has been delineated, and the amino acid composition is similar in the three preparations. There are 84 residual amino acids in PTH, with a total molecular weight of approximately 9500. Biologic activity resides in the initial 30 amino acid residues of the molecule. Synthetic peptides comprising the first 34 amino acids have been produced, and they are biologically active.

PTH is synthesized within the parathyroid gland initially as a prohormone comprising 109 amino acids. Pro-PTH is only about one-half as biologically active as PTH. Conversion of pro-PTH to PTH occurs within the parathyroid cells, producing the 84 residual peptides. Following appropriate physiologic stimulus, PTH is secreted into the circulation and undergoes a second cleavage, perhaps in the liver, into one or more fragments that can be distinguished from the intact hormone by their different immunoreactivity. A large hormonal fragment with a molecular weight of about 7500 appears to be the predominant peptide in the circulation. Both the kidney and the liver contain enzymes that are able to inactivate PTH.

Control of PTH Secretion

Conclusive experimental and clinical evidence indicates that parathyroid secretion is not under nervous or tropic hormone control. Most, if not all, of the recent evidence is consistent with the generally accepted view that the concentration of calcium ion in the blood circulating through the parathyroid gland is the major factor controlling the rate of hormone secretion. A high serum calcium concentration inhibits secretion of PTH, and a low calcium concentration stimulates PTH secretion.

The normal calcium content of the serum varies between 9 and 11 mg/100 ml. Calcium exists in the serum in two forms, the nondiffusible and the diffusible. The nondiffusible part, which represents about 45% of the total serum calcium, is bound to serum protein as calcium proteinate. The diffusible portion is present as calcium carbonate and calcium phosphate. Nearly all of the diffusible calcium is in the ionized form. Only the ionized (diffusible) portion of the calcium is physiologically active, and it is the reduction of ionic calcium that leads to tetany. Dogs with renal disease, with a low serum protein and an associated low serum calcium, do not develop tetany because the reduction is primarily of physiologically inactive, nondiffusible calcium.

The level of calcium in serum depends upon the balance between calcium added from intestinal absorption and bone resorption, and calcium lost from the blood by deposition in the mineral phase of bone and by excretion through the kidney and intestines. The primary function of PTH is to maintain normal extracellular levels of ionized calcium. Thus, as ionized calcium levels decrease in the serum, the parathyroid increases secretion of PTH, which acts mainly upon three target tissues: the gastrointestinal tract, the kidney, and bone.

Although there has been controversy concerning the role of PTH in the regulation of calcium absorption from the gastrointestinal tract, it has been shown that parathyroidectomy decreases calcium absorption, and hyperparathyroidism increases calcium absorption. PTH increases calcium transport in the small intestines, but vitamin D is required for this activity. PTH and vitamin D are synergistic in this action.

Although administration of PTH to parathyroidectomized dogs leads to a rapid increase in urinary excretion of phosphate, sodium, potassium, and bicarbonate, and a decreased excretion of hydrogen ion, ammonia, calcium, and magnesium, most attention has been focused upon the influence of PTH on renal excretion of phosphate. This action occurs within 15 minutes after administration of the hormone. Abundant evidence suggests that the increased phosphate excretion is not mediated through an increase in glomerular filtration rate. In the dog, filtered phosphate normally is reabsorbed in the proximal tubule. PTH increases the rate of phosphate excretion by inhibiting this resorptive mechanism. PTH action is not mediated by a secretory process for phosphate excretion.

The phosphaturic action of PTH is important for the regulation and maintenance of a normal serum calcium concentration. There is a reciprocal relationship between the concentration of serum inorganic phosphorus and the concentration of serum calcium. When a large quantity of inorganic phosphorus is present, the amount of calcium that can be held in solution decreases, and the excess calcium must be eliminated either by excretion into the urine or by deposition into the bone. When a low concentration of inorganic phosphorus is present, a greater amount of calcium can be held in solution. The serum calcium, therefore, varies inversely with the serum phosphorus concentration.

Parathormone has two major and direct effects on bone. It promotes resorption and inhibits formation. Resorption is associated with osteoclastic proliferation and decreased osteoblastic activity. Osteoclasts are capable of absorbing bone, and their activity, which is accompanied by increased alkaline phosphatase activity, can be controlled by either exogenous or endogenous PTH.

Resorption is a complex process involving the destruction of both mineral and matrix. The removal of organic matrix is controlled by PTH in that the hormone induces the synthesis of new enzymes. PTH is unable to enhance calcium mobilization in vitamin D-deficient animals. Thus, it appears that vitamin D is necessary for PTH action on bone.

Calcitonin (CT)

CT is a polypeptide comprising 32 amino acid residues, with a molecular weight of approximately 3500. The source of CT in the *thyroid gland* is the parafollicular cells or C cells that are adjacent to the thyroid follicle. (Immunofluorescent techniques have demonstrated that these cells contain CT.) The evolutionary origin of CT indicates that the parafollicular cells are derived from ultimobranchial tissue. The ultimobranchial body arises from the fifth pharyngeal pouch, and in mammals becomes incorporated into the thyroid gland. The ultimobranchial bodies of the dogfish and chicken contain large quantities of a calcium lowering substance that is believed to be CT.

CT plays an important part in calcium homeostasis by counteracting the effects of PTH. It prevents calcium overshoot and adds greatly to the stability of the serum calcium. There is evidence that CT may be secreted only at times of severe hypercalcemic stress. CT cannot be detected in the serum of normocalcemic animals by present-day bioassay techniques. The hormone can only be detected with infusion of high levels of calcium. It is possible that the hormone may be more important in development and modeling of the skeleton than in maintenance of a normal serum calcium in the adult animal.

CT increases the excretion of calcium and phosphorus in the urine. The CT-induced phosphaturia is not due to the stimulation of the parathyroid glands, since it can be seen in thyroparathyroidectomized animals.

CT causes a rapid decrease in plasma calcium and phosphorus, the calcium reaching its lowest level only one to two hours after CT administration. The induced hypocalcemia is not mainly the result of the increase in renal calcium excretion, since the hormone is still effective in the nephrectomized animal. Moreover, it is not due to an increased loss of calcium in the gut, since CT can produce hypocalcemia after removal of the gastrointestinal tract. Although this evidence eliminates the gastrointestinal tract and the kidney as sole sites of action of CT, it does not exclude them as possible sites of hormone action.

The current hypothesis is that CT primarily inhibits bone resorption; CT also protects the animal from dangerous effects of hypercalcemia. It appears to act rapidly in preventing plasma calcium from going above physiologic levels. The normal stimulus to CT secretion appears to be the concentration of ionic calcium in circulation.

Vitamin D Metabolism and Function

It has been known for many years that vitamin D plays an important role in calcium metabolism. However, only recently have its metabolism to active forms and the feedback regulation of its metabolism been understood. Vitamin D is necessary for normal calcification of bone, and it is an essential homeostatic agent for control of plasma calcium concentration (Fig. 8–1).

Vitamin D_3 (cholecalciferol) is absorbed from food or is produced in the skin in response to ultraviolet radiation. Transported through the circulatory system to the liver, it is converted to 25-hydroxycholecalciferol (25-OHD_3) and then transported to the kidney. A further transformation produces 1,25-dihydroxycholecalciferol (1,25-$(OH)_2$-D_3), considered to be the active and physiologic form of vitamin D.

After vitamin D is absorbed, it becomes associated with a vitamin-D-binding protein that migrates with the alpha globulins. Recently this vitamin D carrier protein has been purified and found to have a molecular weight of 53,000. It seems likely that vitamin D or its metabolites in the blood are normally associated with the vitamin D transport protein.

Without PTH the normal synthesis of 1,25-$(OH)_2$-D_3 probably cannot occur. 1,25-$(OH)_2$-D_3 is the form of vitamin D_3 that is active in increasing the absorption of calcium in the gastrointestinal tract. This hormone also is necessary for normal calcification of bone, and with PTH, it is important for the reabsorption of calcium from bone. 1,25-$(OH)_2$-D_3 acts on both bone and intestine to mobilize calcium from their contents. As the serum calcium level approaches its normal range, PTH secretion decreases, with a resulting decrease in conversion of 25-OH-D_3 to 1,25-$(OH)_2$-D_3.

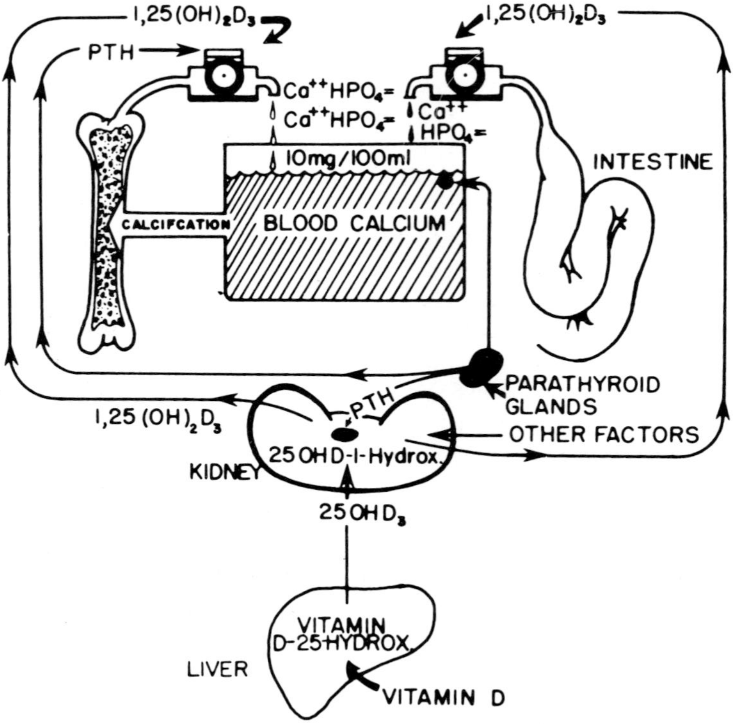

Fig. 8–1. Schematic designation of hormonal control loop for vitamin D metabolism and function. A drop below set point for serum calcium of 10 mg/100 ml prompts a proportional secretion of parathyroid hormone, which acts to increase bone resorption and thus elevates serum calcium. Parathyroid hormone also directs metabolism of 25-OH-D_3 to 1,25-$(OH)_2D_3$ in the kidney, where "hormone" 1,25-$(OH)_2D_3$ acts both on bone and on intestines to mobilize calcium from bone and intestinal contents. As serum calcium increases toward its set point, parathyroid hormone secretion is proportionately decreased. (From Omdahl, J. L., and DeLuca, H. F.: Physiol. Rev., 53:327, 1973.)

HYPOPARATHYROIDISM

The first reported instance of hypoparathyroid tetany in the dog occurred in 1884 when a high percentage of operated dogs died following removal of their "thyroid" glands. Their deaths were described as being accompanied by acute nervous symptoms. Not until 1891 was it revealed that the thyroidectomy performed by the previous investigators had also included removal of the parathyroid glands. An important step in the knowledge of the parathyroid gland function came in 1909 when it was shown that tetany could be produced by destruction of the parathyroid glands themselves. It was then concluded that the parathyroids secreted a material that controlled the calcium exchange in the body, and that an insufficiency or deficiency of calcium at the tissue level resulted in tetany. It was also demonstrated that the parenteral administration of calcium salts into the tetanic animal promptly eliminated all signs and restored the animal to an apparently normal state.

In 1929 a potent extract from parathyroid tissue was isolated. When administered once or twice daily, this material protected the parathyroidectomized dog against tetany. If tetany had already developed in the parathyroidectomized dog, it could be completely relieved by parathyroid extract.

During this time, a close relationship was observed between the clinical condition of the experimental animals and the calcium of the blood serum. The marked improvement observed after use of the active extract coincided with a rise in the blood calcium. It was concluded that the principal effect of this hormone was an increase in calcium content of the blood serum to within its normal limits.

Based upon these experimental parathyroidectomies, the researchers determined that the signs of canine parathormone deprivation are: (1) a fall in serum calcium, (2) a rise in the serum inorganic phosphorus, (3) a decrease in the excretion of urinary calcium, (4) a decrease in the excretion of urinary phosphorus, (5) increased excitability of the musculature to mechanical stimulation, (6) fibrillary twitchings of the muscles followed by jerking muscular contractions, and (7) death usually due to asphyxia secondary to spasms of the laryngeal and thoracic muscles. As serum calcium levels of the blood fall, the symptoms become progressively more severe.

The most common cause of tetany associated with insufficiency of PTH is that encountered secondary to accidental removal of/or injury to the parathyroid glands during thyroidectomy. One remaining parathyroid gland is sufficient to prevent the occurrence of tetany. If clinical signs of tetany improve or disappear within a few days to a few weeks following thyroidectomy, it is assumed that the parathyroid glands were injured during surgery rather than inadvertently removed, and that the injured parathyroid tissue has regained its function. When the clinical signs of tetany remain permanently, it must be assumed that all parathyroid glands were inadvertently removed along with the thyroid.

A rare disease, idiopathic hypoparathyroidism, has been described in man. To my knowledge, it has not been reported in the dog.

Clinical Signs

Usually tetany develops 24 to 96 hours following thyroidectomy, or more correctly thyroparathyroidectomy. Neuromuscular excitability develops, and spasms of the muscles may become so severe that, if uncorrected, will produce convulsions. More commonly, only evidence of hyperexcitability of the muscles is observed. Examination of the blood shows a lowering of the serum calcium to 8 mg/100 ml or below, and a corresponding rise in the serum phosphorus of 4 to 5 mg/100 ml. There is also a decrease in the calcium and phosphate in the urine. The reduction in serum calcium is directly responsible for the neuromuscular hyperexcitability. Laryngeal spasms may occur; if so, they lead to dyspnea.

Treatment

The specific therapy for hypoparathyroidism depends upon whether the acute phase of the disease is occurring, that is, the immediate period following parathyroidectomy; or whether the treatment is directed at the later and more chronic phase following recovery from surgery. In the early or acute phase, treatment is aimed at preventing muscle spasms and convulsions by restoring the serum calcium levels to near normal. Intravenous injection of calcium salts, preferably calcium gluconate, will quickly raise the serum calcium level and relieve the clinical signs. This type of medication should be given to effect. However, treatment with intravenous calcium salts is of short duration, necessitating repeated doses several times during the first 12 to 24 hours to keep the animal free of clinical signs. As soon as possible, calcium per os should be administered. To assure maximum absorption of calcium, sufficient doses of vitamin D should be administered. Satisfactory control is obtained using calcium gluconate or calcium lactate per os and vitamin D. For a 20- to 40-pound dog, 5 g of calcium gluconate and 100,000 IU of vitamin D are usually effective in preventing signs of tetany. The availability of parathyroid extract is limited; therefore, it is not a practical way to treat hypoparathyroidism.

PSEUDOHYPOPARATHYROIDISM

With the development of radioimmunoassay for PTH, additional clinical syndromes have been documented; these syndromes have some aspects in common with hypoparathyroidism. Classically hypoparathyroidism, whether idiopathic or surgically induced, results from failure to secrete PTH. In contrast, pseudohypoparathyroidism is a disease due to an end-organ refractoriness to hormone action. In addition to the usual features of hypoparathyroidism, such as hypocalcemia and tetany, peculiar somatic features have been described in man. Pseudohypoparathyroid individuals generally have shorter metacarpals and metatarsals, tetany, intermittent hypocalcemia, and relative end-organ insensitivity to parathyroid extract.

In one syndrome of man the physical defects of

pseudohypoparathyroidism are present, but the serum calcium and phosphorus concentrations are essentially normal. This disorder is termed *pseudopseudohypoparathyroidism*. Since PTH increases urinary 3′,5′-AMP, it has been possible to differentiate pseudohypoparathyroidism from pseudopseudohypoparathyroidism. In patients with pseudohypoparathyroidism, there is no increase in urinary 3′,5′-AMP in response to PTH administration. In contrast, a normal response occurs in patients with pseudopseudohypoparathyroidism. This difference signifies a lack of or a defect in PTH-sensitive adenyl cyclase in bone and kidney of patients with pseudohypoparathyroidism.

Idiopathic hypoparathyroidism, pseudohypoparathyroidism, and pseudopseudohypoparathyroidism have not been described in the dog. When immunoassay of PTH is more commonly utilized in canine medicine, these disorders will probably be recognized.

PRIMARY HYPERPARATHYROIDISM

Excessive secretion of PTH may be caused by one or more benign tumors in separate parathyroid glands (Fig. 8–2), a malignant tumor of one gland, or hyperplasia of all four glands. Primary hyper-

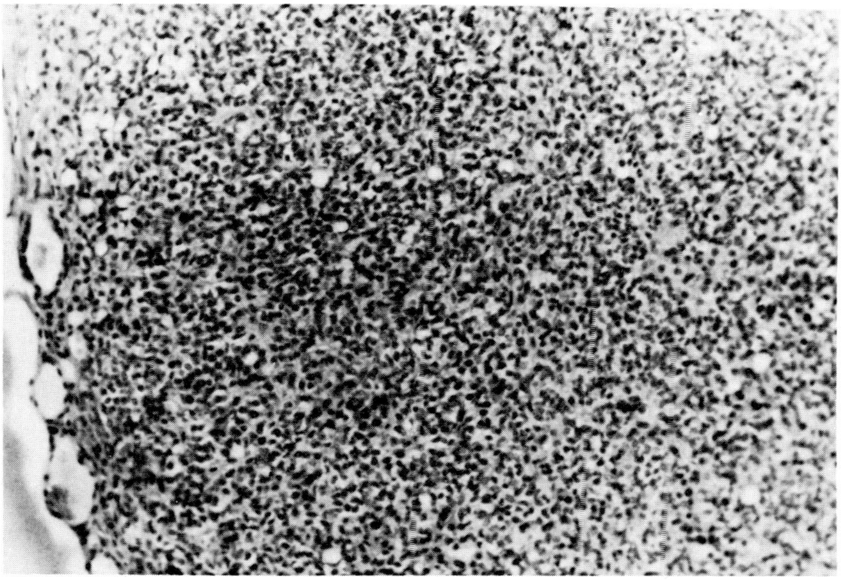

Fig. 8–2. Parathyroid adenoma ×102. Solid tumor containing occasional foci with differentiation to "chief-like" cells. (Courtesy John T. McGrath, University of Pennsylvania.)

parathyroidism involves excessive secretion of PTH, and the primary pathologic changes reside within the parathyroid tissue itself. This disorder is a disease of extreme variation, both in severity and in mode of clinical expression. It may be completely asymptomatic, or it may show extensive involvement of the skeletal and/or urinary system. Hypercalcemia is the one most important criterion necessary for diagnosis. Nevertheless, the serum calcium level may also be borderline, equivocal, or occasionally normal.

Detection of primary hyperparathyroidism has been hampered by the inadequacy of diagnostic tests. No single test, other than radioimmunoassay of PTH, positively confirms or excludes the diagnosis of primary hyperparathyroidism. In most circumstances, the state of parathyroid function is evaluated by the changes in metabolic processes known to be influenced by PTH, in essence, by alterations in plasma and urinary calcium and inorganic phosphorus levels.

Clinical Signs

Hypercalcemia due to primary hyperparathyroidism must be differentiated from hypercalcemia due to other disorders, such as vitamin D intoxication, adrenal insufficiency, thyrotoxicosis, immobilization, and malignant diseases. Patients with certain carcinomas may present exceptional diagnostic problems, not only because they have hypercalcemia and hypophosphatemia, but also because their tumors may actually secrete a peptide that is similar, if not identical, to PTH.

Although the single most important diagnostic feature of primary hyperparathyroidism is hypercalcemia, this symptom may be intermittent rather than constant. Hypophosphatemia was once considered an important diagnostic feature of this disease, but increasing experience in human medicine has shown that serum phosphorus has only limited usefulness in the differential diagnosis. Hypophosphatemia is common in hyperparathyroidism, but it may also be absent.

Plasma alkaline phosphatase values increase with primary hyperparathyroidism only when bone disease is present. Despite experimental evidence that virtually all affected individuals have increased bone mineral turnover rates, plasma alkaline phosphatase elevations are usually noted only in those individuals with specific radiographic signs of hyperparathyroidism, such as bone "cysts" or subperiosteal resorption.

Hyperparathyroidism is further complicated by its occasional ability to cause unequivocal end-organ damage, such as osteitis fibrosa cystica and/or nephrocalcinosis. At other times the only symptom may be hypercalcemia without evidence of any end-organ damage. In the dog, hyperparathyroidism is usually recognized when it is associated with end-organ damage. Despite its remarkable variability, primary hyperparathyroidism is considered a single clinical entity in which the principal clinical features reflect primary differences in duration or severity of hormone excess. Despite the high incidence of this condition in man, the more severe manifestations of the disease, i.e., generalized osteitis fibrosa cystica and hypercalcemic crisis, remain relative rarities.

Clinical signs seen with symptomatic primary hyperparathyroidism are essentially those related to the elevated serum calcium level. If hypercalcemia is advanced, anorexia, depression, weakness, polyuria, emesis, and dehydration are present.

Classically, hypercalcemia, hypercalciuria, and hypophosphatemia have been cardinal signs suggesting an increased PTH secretion. However, since some of these findings are inconsistent, the final diagnosis depends upon the demonstration of increased PTH secretion. The diagnosis can be further confused since PTH can be secreted by malignant tumors of nonparathyroid tissue. With malignant tumors producing PTH or PTH-like material, the hypercalcemia may be reduced by administration of cortisol or equivalent steroid therapy. In primary hyperparathyroidism, steroids do not decrease the hypercalcemia. Some clinicians have seen this response to therapeutic administration of steroids, and have advocated steroids as an aid to the differential diagnosis of hypercalcemia. The specificity of the "steroid test" has been questioned by other investigators; they report that effective preoperative suppression of hypercalcemia is observed in some instances of proven hyperparathyroidism. In addition, a lack of response in patients with hypercalcemia of nonparathyroid origin has occasionally been reported. The steroid suppression test must be interpreted with extreme care.

Hypercalcemic Crisis

Occasionally a life-threatening hypercalcemic crisis may develop, frequently accompanied by polyuria, polydipsia, and profound weakness. Rapidly progressive renal failure and cardiovascular collapse may occur terminally. In this desperate situation, many methods for reducing serum calcium have been tried. Intravenous administration of the disodium salt of edathanil (EDTA), a chelating agent, is not favored because it may have an adverse effect on renal function, already seriously impaired. Massive water loading with administration of furosemide to produce maximal diuresis is perhaps one of the safer and more effective regimens available.

At present, surgical removal of a parathyroid tumor or subtotal resection of hyperplastic parathyroid glands is the only effective therapy for primary hyperparathyroidism. Following this procedure, normal calcium levels promptly return, and other biochemical abnormalities eventually disappear. With the diagnosis of primary hyperparathyroidism, even surgical exploration occasionally must be done as a confirming diagnostic maneuver. The parathyroid adenoma may be quite small, so the diagnosis may be difficult even at the time of the surgical procedure. In the majority of cases, surgical extirpation provides satisfactory cure of primary hyperparathyroidism.

Parathyroprivic tetany is usually the most serious possible consequence of surgery though its incidence is rare. If tetany does develop following surgery, it is usually self-limited since the remaining parathyroid tissue will regain its function. However, full function of the remaining parathyroid tissue may take as long as a few weeks. Vigorous treatment with calcium and vitamin D should be avoided, since most affected individuals can tolerate minimal hypocalcemia. Furthermore, the hypocalcemia stimulates the remaining parathyroid tissue to regain normal function. Any excessive treatment of the hypocalcemia will delay the return of normal parathyroid function.

The diagnosis of primary hyperparathyroidism is accomplished by correlating clinical findings with simple laboratory determinations. Until a reliable technique for measurement of canine PTH is available, the clinician will have to utilize routine serum calcium screenings and other appropriate indirect testing procedures to arrive at a diagnosis. Hypercalcemia is the hallmark of the disease, and the diagnosis involves predominantly the differentiation between hyperparathyroidism and other diseases that can give rise to hypercalcemia.

SECONDARY HYPERPARATHYROIDISM

Any abnormality that decreases the serum calcium concentration stimulates the parathyroid glands. Its response to this decrease produces secondary hyperparathyroidism. A number of disorders can produce a secondary increase in PTH secretion, including excessive cortisol secretion with Cushing's syndrome, hyperphosphatemia associated with renal insufficiency, pseudohypoparathyroidism, vitamin D deficiency, hypercalcitonemia associated with medullary carcinoma of the thyroid gland, and nutritional hyperparathyroidism associated with feeding an all meat diet containing an unfavorable calcium to phosphorus ratio.

Secondary hyperparathyroidism is always associated with diffuse hyperplasia and enlargement of all parathyroid glands. It occurs as a result of an increased demand on the parathyroids. Most commonly, it is associated with chronic renal insufficiency with hyperphosphatemia. The hyperphosphatemia depresses the circulating level of calcium, thus stimulating parathyroid activity, which in turn increases the blood calcium level. The chief importance of secondary hyperparathyroidism is its occurrence in association with hypocalcemic disorders.

TERTIARY HYPERPARATHYROIDISM

Protracted stimulation of the parathyroid glands leads to tertiary hyperparathyroidism, in which the glands secrete autonomously. It may develop in individuals with renal disorders; when it does, both hypercalcemia and hyperphosphatemia are present. The importance of this disorder lies in its conversion of a secondary hyperparathyroidism into one that has true autonomy.

PSEUDOHYPERPARATHYROIDISM

Secretion of PTH by tumors of nonparathyroid tissue produces the syndrome of pseudohyperparathyroidism. This disorder has been

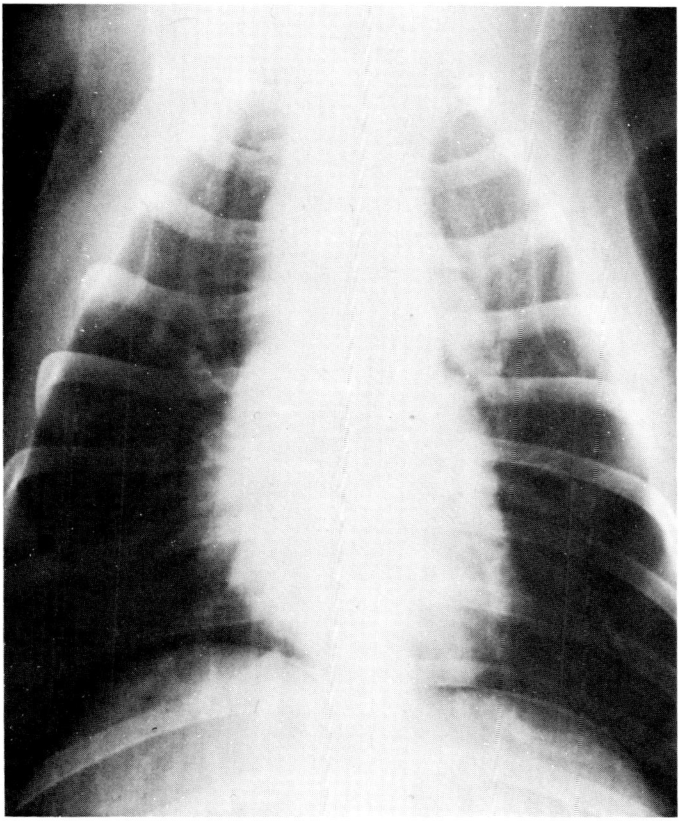

Fig. 8–3. Female Weimaraner (7½ years of age) with pseudohyperparathyroidism. An anterior mediastinal mass is present which was found to be lymphosarcoma.

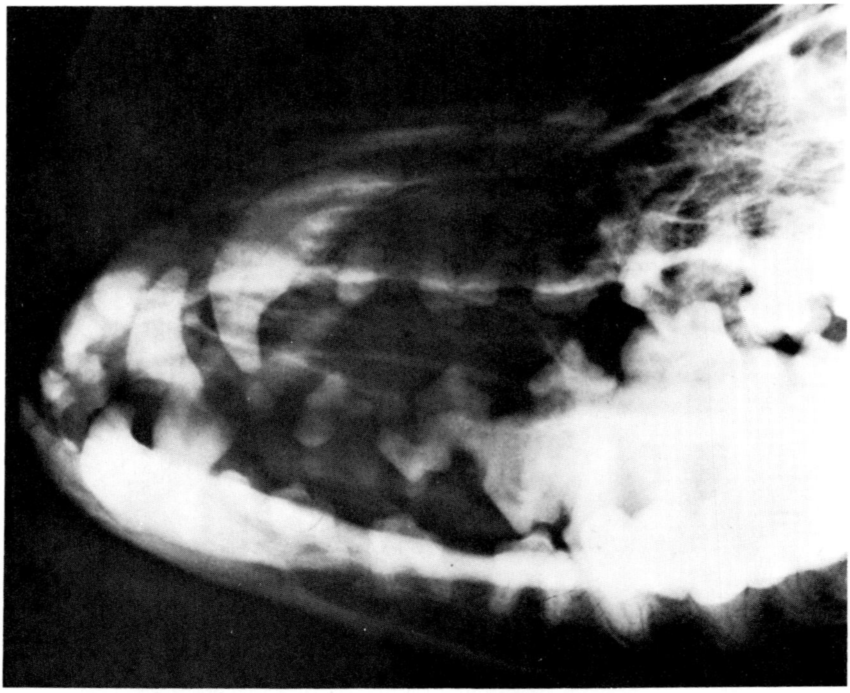

Fig. 8–4. Roentgenogram of the head of the animal described in Fig. 8–3. There is marked demineralization with loss of the lamina dura.

described in man with many different types of neoplasms. At present it has been reported in the dog only with lymphatic-type tumors, i.e., lymphosarcoma (Fig. 8–3). The secretion of PTH or PTH-like material by these tumors creates a hyperparathyroid-like syndrome with all of the clinical findings of primary hyperparathyroidism (Fig. 8–4). As described earlier in this chapter, pseudohyperparathyroidism can occasionally be differentiated from primary hyperparathyroidism by utilizing a cortisol suppression test. The hypercalcemia of pseudohyperparathyroidism is more responsive to therapeutic levels of steroids than is the hypercalcemia of primary hyperparathyroidism.

SELECTED READING

1. Anglem, T. J.: Acute hyperparathyroidism: a surgical emergency. Surg. Clin. North Am., *46*:727, 1966.
2. Arnaud, C. D., Jr., Tenenhouse, A. M., and Rasmussen, H.: Parathyroid hormone. Annu. Rev. Physiol., *29*:349, 1967.
3. Avioli, L. V.: The diagnosis of primary hyperparathyroidism. Med. Clin. North Am., *52*:451, 1968.

4. Bartlett, W. C.: Acute hyperparathyroid crisis. Am. J. Surg., *114*:796, 1967.
5. Borle, A. B.: Calcium and phosphate metabolism. Annu. Rev. Physiol., *36*:361, 1974.
6. Bramley, P., and Dwyer, D.: Primary hyperparathyroidism. Oral Surg., *30*:464, 1970.
7. Burkhart, J. M., and Jowsey, J.: Morphologic evidence of osteomalacia in the parathyroidectomized dog. Mayo Clin. Proc., *41*:663, 1966.
8. Chopra, I. J., and Nugent, C. A.: Concurrence of features of pseudohypoparathyroidism, pseudopseudohypoparathyroidism and basal-cell nevus syndrome. Am. J. Med. Sc., *260*:171, 1970.
9. Cramer, C. F.: Participation of parathyroid glands in control of calcium absorption in dogs. Endocrinology, *72*:192, 1963.
10. DeLuca, H. F.: The kidney as an endocrine organ for the production of 1,25-dihydroxyvitamin D_3, a calcium-mobilizing hormone. N. Engl. J. Med., *289*:359, 1973.
11. Dimich, A., Bedrossian, P. B., and Wallach, S.: Hypoparathyroidism. Arch. Intern. Med., *120*:449, 1967.
12. Epstein, F. H.: Calcium and the kidney. Am. J. Med., *45*:700, 1968.
13. Fasnacht, D. W., and Maksic, D.: Primary hyperparathyroidism in a dog. Mod. Vet. Pract., *43*:38, 1962.
14. Gale, T. C., and Owens, C. W. I.: Hyperfunctioning carcinoma of the parathyroid gland. Postgrad. Med. J., *48*:626, 1972.
15. Goldman, L., and Greenspan, F. S.: Applied physiology of the thyroid and parathyroid glands. Surg. Clin. North Am., *45*:317, 1965.
16. Goldsmith, R. E., Wulsin, J., and Wiester, M. J.: Effect of thyroparathyroidectomy on the clinical course and the serum calcium and phosphorus concentration in dogs. Endocrinology, *76*:9, 1965.
17. Hodges, M., and Waterhouse, C.: Hypercalcemia of hyperparathyroidism responsive to prednisone. Arch. Intern. Med., *120*:75, 1967.
18. Keating, F. R., Jr.: The clinical problem of primary hyperparathyroidism. Med. Clin. North Am., *54*:511, 1970.
19. Kirk, G. R., Breazile, J. E., and Kenny, A. D.: Pathogenesis of hypocalcemic tetany in the thyroparathyroidectomized dog. Am. J. Vet. Res., *35*:407, 1974.
20. Klopper, P. J., and Moe, R. E.: Demonstration of the parathyroids during surgery in dogs, with preliminary report of results in some clinical cases. Surgery, *59*:1101, 1966.
21. Kraintz, L.: A new view of parathyroid and thyroid physiology in relation to calcium metabolism. J. Oral Ther. Pharmacol., *2*:270, 1966.
22. Krook, L.: Spontaneous hyperparathyroidism in the dog. Acta Pathol. Microbiol. Scand. [Suppl. 122], *41*:27, 1958.
23. MacLeod, W. A. J., and Holloway, C. K.: Hyperparathyroid crisis. Ann. Surg., *166*:1012, 1967.
24. Munson, P. L., Hirsch, P. F., and Tashjian, A. H.: Parathyroid gland. Annu. Rev. Physiol., *25*:325, 1963.
25. Normann, E., Seljelid, R., and Nakken, K. F.: Uptake of ^{3}H-labelled toluidine blue and neutral red in the parathyroids of the dog. Scand. J. Clin. Lab. Invest., *26*:369, 1970.
26. Nusynowitz, M. L., and Klein, M. H.: Pseudoidiopathic hypoparathyroidism. Am. J. Med., *55*:677, 1973.
27. Omdahl, J. L., and DeLuca, H. F.: Regulation of vitamin D metabolism and function. Physiol. Rev., *53*:327, 1973
28. Osborne, C. A., and Stevens, J. B.: Pseudohyperparathyroidism in the dog. J. Am. Vet. Med. Assoc., *162*:125, 1973.
29. Pak, C. Y. C.: Parathyroid hormone and thyrocalcitonin: their mode of action and regulation. Ann. N. Y. Acad. Sci., *179*:450, 1971.
30. Pearson, P. T., et al.: Primary hyperparathyroidism in a beagle. J. Am. Vet. Med. Assoc., *147*:1201, 1965.
31. Pittinger, C., Chang, P. M., and Faulkner, W.: Serum ionized calcium. South. Med. J., *64*:1211, 1971.
32. Rasmussen, H.: Secondary hyperparathyroidism. Mt. Sinai J. Med. N. Y., *40*:462, 1973.

33. Reiss, E.: Primary hyperparathyroidism: a simplified approach to diagnosis. Med. Clin. North Am., *54*:131, 1970.
34. Renk, W.: Epithelkörperchen-Glandulae Parathyroidales. Handbuch der speziellen pathologischen Anatomie der Haustiere, Verlag P. Parey, Berlin, *3*:89, 1962.
35. Roth, S. I.: Recent advances in parathyroid gland pathology. Am. J. Med., *50*:612, 1971.
36. Roy, C. C., and O'Brien, D.: Calcium and phosphorus current concepts of metabolism. Clin. Pediat., *6*:19, 1967.
37. Samaan, N. A., Hickey, R. C., Hill, C. S., Jr., Medellin, H., and Gates, R. B.: Parathyroid tumors: preoperative localization and association with other tumors. Cancer, *33*:933, 1974.
38. Samiy, A. H., Hirsch, P. F., and Ramsay, A. G.: Localization of phosphaturic effect of parathyroid hormone in nephron of the dog. Am. J. Physiol., *208*:73, 1965.
39. Saville, P. D., et al.: Nutritional secondary hyperparathyroidism in a dog. Morphologic and radioisotope studies with treatment. Cornell Vet., *59*:155, 1969.
40. Sherwood, L. M.: Relative importance of parathyroid hormone and thyrocalcitonin in calcium homeostasis. N. Engl. J. Med., *278*:663, 1968.
41. Stavrou, D.: Beitrag zum Hyperparathyroidismus des Hundes. Deutsche tierarztl. Wchnschr., *75*:117, 1968.
42. Tenenhouse, A., Rasmussen, H., Hawker, C. D., and Arnaud, C. D.: Thyrocalcitonin. Annu. Rev. Pharmacol., *8*:319, 1968.
43. Treusch, J. V., and Cohen, S.: Idiopathic hypoparathyroidism follow-up study including autopsy findings of a case previously reported. Ann. Intern. Med., *56*:484, 1962.
44. Taylor, D. M., and Siemsen, A. W.: Bronchogenic carcinoma simulating hyperparathyroidism. Arch. Intern. Med., *115*:67, 1965.
45. Wasserman, R. H.: Metabolism, function and clinical aspects of vitamin D. Cornell Vet., *65*:1, 1975.
46. Wagner, D. H.: The function of the parathyroid glands and their disturbances. Surg. Clin. North Am., *42*:171, 1962.
47. Wibell, L., Johansson, H., and Werner, I.: The use of a calcium infusion test in the diagnosis of hyperparathyroidism. Scand. J. Clin. Lab. Invest., *30*:183, 1972.
48. Wilson, J. W., Harris, S. G., Moore, W. D., and Leipold, H. W.: Primary hyperparathyroidism in a dog. J. Am. Vet. Med. Assoc., *164*:942, 1974.

Chapter 9

The Pancreas

Functionally the pancreas comprises two separate glands, one exocrine, the other endocrine. The exocrine secretions contain digestive enzymes, and are transported into the gastrointestinal tract by one or more ducts. The secretory unit is the acinus, a collection of cells containing zymogen granules. The endocrine function of the pancreas is contained within the islets of Langerhans, and the main hormones secreted are insulin and glucagon.

ANATOMY

The pancreas is a rather coarsely lobulated and elongated pinkish-grey gland. In the dog it is essentially a V-shaped structure with the right lobe lying close to the duodenum. The right lobe runs cranially toward the pylorus where it forms the pancreatic angle, the area uniting the two lobes. The left lobe lies within the greater omentum along the greater curvature of the stomach. It is about two-thirds as long and half again as wide as the right lobe.

Histologically, several cell types can be distinguished in the islets of Langerhans. The two main granulated cell types are the alpha and beta cells. The alpha cells are responsible for the secretion of glucagon, whereas the beta cells secrete insulin. Occasionally accessory pancreatic tissue is seen in the dog. The ectopic locations described are the wall of the gall bladder and the caudal part of the great mesentery.

PHYSIOLOGY

Proinsulin and Insulin

Proinsulin, a single polypeptide-chain precursor of insulin, is produced in the beta cells of the islets of Langerhans. It has little biologic activity. Proinsulin contains the A and B chains of insulin linked by a polypeptide segment of approximately 30 amino acids (Fig. 9–1). Conversion of proinsulin to insulin also occurs in the beta cells. The structures of porcine and bovine proinsulins are known; they have considerable differences in the sequence of their connecting segments. The structure of canine proinsulin has not been determined as yet. The amino acid composition of insulin has been determined in a variety of mammalian species. Canine insulin is identical to pig, sperm whale, and fin whale insulin.

The route of glucose ingestion, as well as its concentration in blood, is important in stimulating insulin secretion. Higher levels of circulating insulin are observed following an oral glucose load than after an equivalent intravenous dose. As glucose contacts the gastrointestinal mucosa, there is a release of gastrointestinal hormones that augment insulin secretion. Current evidence suggests that secretin and gastrointestinal glucagon play a physiologic role in this enhanced insulin secretion. Gastrointestinal glucagon is a polypeptide that chemically and immunologically resembles pancreatic glucagon, but does not have the gluconeogenic and glycogenolytic properties of the hormone produced by the pancreatic alpha cells.

In addition to glucose, amino acids are also capable of stimulating insulin secretion. Pure protein feeding gives rise to increased insulin secretion. Gastrointestinal factors probably play a role in this mechanism. Individual amino acids vary in their capacity to stimulate increased insulin secretion, but virtually all essential amino acids are effective in this mechanism.

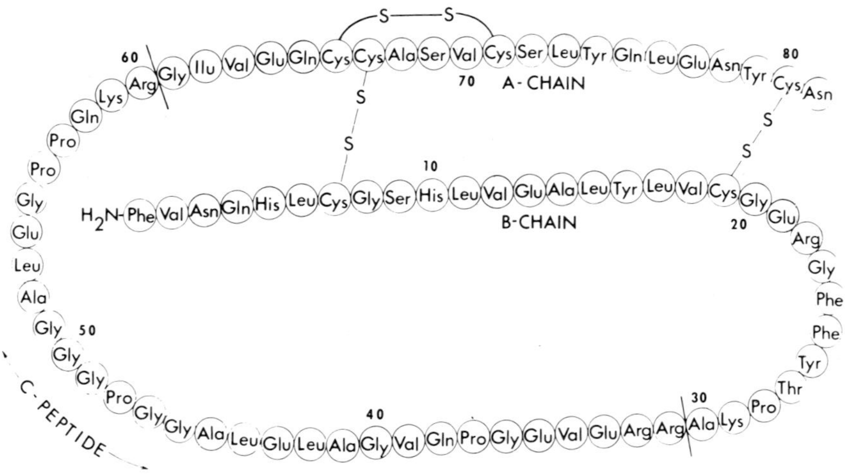

Fig. 9–1. Structure of bovine proinsulin. (From Rubenstein, A. H.: Med. Clin. North Am., *54*:191, 1970.)

Although glucose is the major stimulus for insulin secretion in many species, other physiologic substances are important in this mechanism in specific isolated species. For example, fatty acids exert a marked effect on insulin secretion in ruminants, and amino acids appear to serve as the major stimulus for insulin secretion in fish. In addition, some people appear to have an increased sensitivity to certain amino acids in that hypoglycemia may follow their ingestion. For example, leucine-induced hypoglycemia is a fall in blood glucose associated with leucine ingestion. This amino acid stimulates a hypersecretion in blood insulin levels in affected individuals. In the dog, besides glucose and amino acids, aceto-acetate, beta-hydroxybutyrate, and free fatty acids have all been shown to stimulate the secretion of insulin.

Metabolic Effects of Insulin

The pronounced effect of insulin on carbohydrate homeostasis often focuses attention upon this important function. However, insulin is also intimately involved in the metabolism of fat and protein. Insulin functions as the prime hormone expediting the conservation of major metabolic fuels within the body. This regulation of metabolic processes by insulin is essentially carried out in three tissues: the liver, adipose tissue, and skeletal muscle.

Although insulin increases transport of glucose into adipose and muscle cells, insulin is not necessary for entry of glucose into all cells. The membranes of liver cells are freely permeable to glucose; thus, insulin acts upon the liver not to promote glucose uptake, but to suppress intracellular processes involved in glucose production and release. This suppression occurs by altering enzyme activity rather than by influencing membrane transport.

The liver is quantitatively the major site of disposal of ingested glucose. When glucose is consumed, the major proportion is disposed of by the liver, with only about one-third reaching the extrahepatic tissues. The liver possesses an enzyme that converts glucose to glucose-6-phosphate. In the presence of glucose and insulin, this enzyme's activity is enhanced. Insulin also stimulates a second enzyme, which promotes conversion of most of the phosphorylated glucose to glycogen.

The liver also is capable of gluconeogenesis, i.e., formation of new glucose. Insulin suppresses key enzymes and cofactors involved in gluconeogenesis. Insulin also acts to inhibit glycogen breakdown by promoting inactivation of the enzyme required for release of glucose from glycogen. The net effect of these actions is the storage of glucose in the form of glycogen.

In contrast to liver, adipose tissue is unable to take up glucose in the absence of insulin. Insulin increases the permeability of the fat cell membrane to glucose. By virtue of its action on glucose metabolism, insulin has a dual effect in enhancing fat accumulation. It provides precursors for fatty acid synthesis and glycerol for esterification in storage of these fatty acids as triglycerides. In addition, insulin is extremely effective in inhibiting a fat-cell enzyme that catalyzes hydrolysis of stored triglycerides and liberation of free fatty acids. This antilipolytic action of insulin occurs at concentrations that are below those necessary to effect glucose transport. The net effect of the fat-synthetic, glycerogenic, and antilipolytic actions of insulin is increased total fat storage, with conversion of energy ingested in the form of carbohydrates to a more compact storage form, lipid.

As in adipose tissue, insulin is necessary for the transport of glucose across the muscle cell membrane. Glucose taken up by the muscle cell is metabolized to either lactate or carbon dioxide, or it is converted to glycogen. Glucose uptake by muscle in the postabsorptive state accounts for little of the total muscle fuel requirements. With exercise, total glucose utilization may increase tenfold or more above basal levels. This exercise-induced augmentation of glucose utilization is not insulin dependent. In fact it accounts for the frequent diminution of insulin requirements and the tendency towards hypoglycemia observed in insulin-treated diabetics whose activity has been appreciably increased.

Insulin stimulates the uptake of amino acids and their incorporation into muscle protein. This anabolic action of insulin is essential in that growth hormone will not elicit a positive protein balance in the absence of insulin.

These diverse metabolic effects of insulin are integrated and synergistic. Inhibition of hepatic gluconeogenesis decreases the requirements of the liver for amino acids. The anabolic action of insulin reduces the output of amino acids from muscle, diminishing their availability for hepatic gluconeogenesis. At the same time, amino acid incorporation into muscle protein is facilitated. Glucose uptake by muscle is also stimulated, providing an energy source to replace fatty acids whose release from adipose tissue is greatly inhibited by the antilipolytic action. Finally, the antilipolytic action of insulin reinforces the inhibition of hepatic gluconeogenesis by depriving the liver of an energy source (fatty acids) and cofactors (acetyl CoA) vital to the gluconeogenesis process.

Insulin and Other Hormones

Administration of anterior pituitary extracts or purified growth hormone to mature dogs over prolonged periods produces permanent diabetes. Growth hormone has a direct effect on insulin secretion in that high circulating levels of growth hormone, whether produced by exogenous administration or by endogenous secretion, are accompanied by increased serum insulin levels. One explanation of the pathogenesis of growth-hormone-induced diabetes is that prolonged administration of growth hormone initially stimulates hypersecretion of insulin. As this condition progresses, the pancreas is unable to continue this high level of secretion. The development of permanent diabetes occurs after the fall in insulin secretion as the pancreas enters into a phase of "exhaustion atrophy."

At normal and physiologic concentrations, plasma levels of insulin and growth hormone have an inverse relationship. After ingestion of glucose, the plasma level of insulin increases, while growth hormone levels tend to fall. During fasting or prolonged starvation, low plasma levels of insulin and high levels of growth hormone are observed. Both growth hormone and insulin appear to be regulated in response to the glucose concentration in serum or plasma. One chemical test used to assess growth hormone secretion is based on the fact that insulin-induced hypoglycemia stimulates growth hormone secretion.

Glucocorticoids alter insulin secretion indirectly through their action on gluconeogenesis. Higher than normal concentrations of corticosteroids, as seen in dogs with Cushing's syndrome or in dogs receiving therapeutic doses of glucocorticoids, lead to an elevated insulin secretion (Fig. 9–2). This increase has been shown to be secondary to the increase in gluconeogenesis. Early in the course of Cushing's syndrome, or whenever glucocorticoids are administered

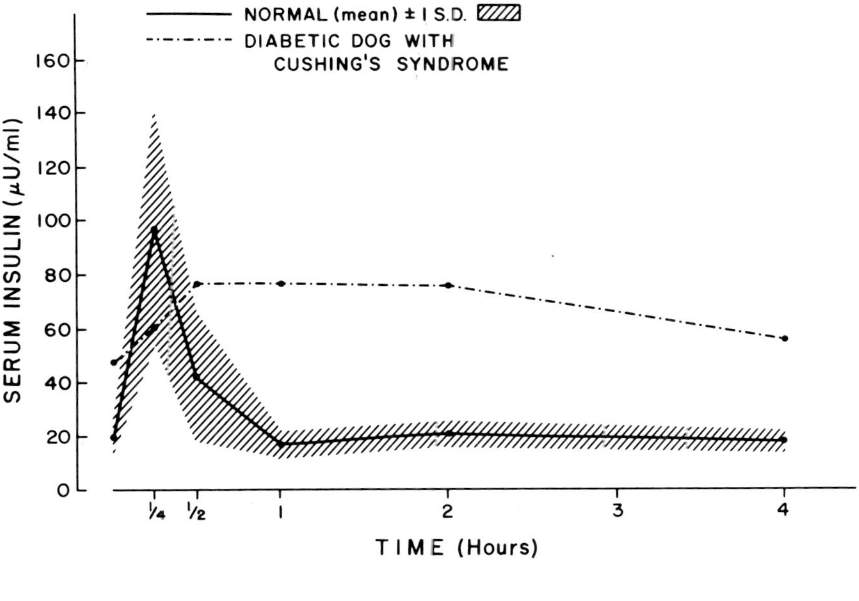

Fig. 9–2. Serum insulin levels in a dog with Cushing's syndrome and secondary diabetes mellitus.

acutely, the blood glucose does not become elevated in the dog, since the increased gluconeogenesis stimulates a compensatory increase in insulin secretion, which tends to maintain the glucose level within the normal range. Following prolonged and excessive secretion or administration of glucocorticoids, the pancreas may be unable to keep up with this increased insulin demand. Then the blood glucose level will become elevated, and a steroid-induced diabetes may result.

Glucagon produces an increase in the blood glucose level and, therefore, has an indirect effect on insulin secretion. However, a more important effect of glucagon is that it stimulates insulin release directly. This stimulation precedes any increase in blood sugar level.

Thyroxine affects glucose homeostasis in a number of ways that can indirectly alter insulin secretion. Thyroxine increases blood sugar levels by increasing the absorption of carbohydrates in the intestinal tract, by increasing glycogenolysis in the liver, and by favoring gluconeogenesis. These actions, which produce an increased blood glucose level, are followed by increased insulin secretion. Epinephrine directly inhibits insulin secretion, and induces hyperglycemia by increasing hepatic glycogenolysis. If epinephrine did not have a direct inhibitory effect on insulin secretion, the resulting hyperglycemia would be followed by a compensatory increase in insulin, which would dampen any increase in blood glucose concentration. Epinephrine inhibits insulin secretion at the same time that it is stimulating hepatic glycogenolysis. These actions are synergistic and produce an elevated blood glucose level.

Glucagon

Glucagon was discovered in a rather inauspicious way as a contaminant of commercial insulin. During some of the early experiments with insulin, researchers found that injection of newly prepared pancreatic extracts into diabetic dogs produced, in addition to the expected hypoglycemia, a rapid and short-lived hyperglycemia. This paradoxic effect was due to a contaminant, which was later called glucagon. In the past the physiologic role of glucagon has been rather elusive. With the advent of sensitive radioimmunoassay, it has become possible to quantitate minute amounts of glucagon in biologic fluids.

The alpha cells of the islets of Langerhans produce glucagon. This peptide hormone consists of 29 amino acids and has a molecular weight of 3400. The hyperglycemic effect occurs because glucagon can increase hepatic glucose output secondary to stimulation of 3′-5′-AMP formation, activation of hepatic phosphorylase, and ensuing glycogenolysis. Glucagon is also gluconeogenic, and it lowers plasma amino acids and stimulates hepatic conversion of amino acids to glucose and glycogen. Glucagon appears to be lipolytic, but in vivo this effect is largely masked by the lipogenic effect of insulin secreted in response to the hyperglycemia and the insulinosecretory action of glucagon.

A material in extracts of stomach and intestinal mucosa, gastrointestinal glucagon, is immunologically similar to pancreatic glucagon. This substance possesses some, but not all, of the biologic activities of pancreatic glucagon. Gastrointestinal glucagon is secreted in response to oral glucose. This glucagon release by the gastrointestinal tract allows an early release of insulin at meal time. Without having to wait for alimentary hyperglycemia to act as an initial stimulus to insulin release, the timely enterohormonal-stimulated release of insulin provides more appropriate hepatic storage, peripheral dispersion, and utilization of absorbed nutrients. Although gastrointestinal glucagon appears to be of prime importance in the stimulation of pancreatic insulin secretion in response to eating, several other gastrointestinal hormones also appear to be involved in this mechanism. Gastrin, secretin, and pancreozymin, as well as gastrointestinal glucagon, stimulate insulin release. Thus, a complex spectrum of interplay exists between the gastrointestinal system and the islets of Langerhans.

The principal and most rapid action of pancreatic glucagon is elevation of the blood glucose. It increases glycogen breakdown in the liver in a matter of one to two minutes. Oral doses of glucose stimulate a transient rise in glucagon secretion, whereas glucose administered intravenously has no such effect. Gastrointestinal glucagon stimulates insulin secretion, but does not have any of the other classic actions of glucagon. It does not stimulate the breakdown of glycogen or raise the blood glucose.

Regulation of Glucagon Secretion

Glucose taken by mouth results in a rapid, transient rise in gastrointestinal glucagon, which in turn stimulates insulin secretion. Conversely, a rise in blood glucose actively inhibits pancreatic glucagon secretion. Amino acids taken orally or injected intravenously will also increase plasma glucagon. In the case of amino acids the increase is essentially that of pancreatic glucagon. When amino acids are taken orally, the increase in plasma glucagon occurs even before any increase in the level of plasma amino acids. This finding suggests that some material is stimulated by oral administration of amino acids, and that this material in turn mediates the increase in pancreatic glucagon. It is believed that a gastrointestinal hormone, pancreozymin,* is the mediator or stimulator of this pancreatic glucagon. Pancreozymin is known to be stimulated by amino acids and is also known to stimulate pancreatic glucagon secretion.

During fasting or hypoglycemia, pancreatic glucagon secretion is increased. It is probable that growth hormone also stimulates pancreatic glucagon secretion. An elevation of glucagon during fasting enhances glycogen breakdown and gluconeogenesis, tending to keep the blood glucose at the desired level. In addition, since glucagon is lipolytic, during fasting it helps mobilize free fatty acids from adipose tissue as a source of energy.

Physiologic Role of Glucagon

The major function of glucagon is the mobilization of nutrients in time of metabolic need. Many of the effects of glucagon are essentially opposite those of insulin.

During fasting or periods of increased metabolic needs, the secretion of glucagon and epinephrine is stimulated, with a resultant increase of glycogenolysis, gluconeogenesis, and lipolysis. The free fatty acids and epinephrine inhibit glucose utilization and insulin action. Thus, when glucagon is adequately secreted, glucose is effectively spared from being metabolized in insulin-dependent tissues.

Whenever food is readily available, glucose in the diet is absorbed into the bloodstream and inhibits pancreatic glucagon secretion as well as epinephrine secretion. During these periods, insulin is stimulated not only by the hyperglycemia, but also by the gastrointestinal glucagon secretion. At this time, when blood glucose levels are high, gluconeogenesis, glycogenolysis, and lipolysis are suppressed.

Glucagon and Other Hormones

Both pancreatic and gastrointestinal glucagon stimulate insulin secretion. Pancreatic glucagon also stimulates the release of adrenal medullary catecholamines, and catecholamines in turn inhibit insulin secretion. In addition, glucagon, the parathyroids, and calcium metabolism appear to be related. Chronic administration of zinc glucagon produces parathyroid hyperplasia. Hyperparathyroidism and pancreatitis have been reported in man along with an associated hyperglucagonemia. Additionally, during experimental pancreatitis in dogs, hyperglucagonemia has been observed. This condition has been reported in certain human patients with acute pancreatitis. It is not known whether the pancreatitis associated with coexistent hyperparathyroidism is the result of chronic hypercalcemia, or whether hyperglucagonemia associated with primary pancreatitis is responsible for parathyroid hyperplasia.

Glucagon is known to induce hypercalciuria and hypocalcemia particularly in hypercalcemic patients. Glucagon also appears to reduce serum calcium concentrations by blocking reabsorption of bone. It has been suggested that increased glucagon release is responsible for the hypocalcemia of acute pancreatitis. Although glucagon does promote hypercalciuria, recent reports suggest that its calcium-lowering effect is directly related to the release of the calcium-lowering peptide, calcitonin.

LABORATORY TESTS

Pancreatic function is intimately involved with glucose homeostasis. However, a single blood glucose determination represents only an instant evaluation of the blood glucose. It is more thorough to use further detailed tests for determining whether there is any abnormality in carbohydrate homeostasis.

A number of different tolerance tests have been developed to evaluate glucose homeostasis. However, various factors may influence the results of some of the different tolerance tests. First, a number of technical variables, such as glucose dose, the route of glucose administration, the time of the last meal, the time of blood sampling, and the specific glucose analytic procedure used, may influence the results. In addition, several other variables may need to be considered, for example, dietary preparation for the test, any activity permitted during the test, any other associated endocrinopathy, drugs being administered, illness or other stresses, pregnancy, age, and sex. Since all these variables may influence the results of a specific tolerance test, they should be kept as constant as possible in order to have statistically valid results.

Oral Glucose Tolerance Test (OGTT)

The standard amount of glucose administered for the OGTT is 1 g of glucose per pound of body weight. The dose is administered in either a 20 or 50% dextrose solution. Blood samples are taken during fasting (just before administration of glucose), and at one-half, one, two, and four hours after ingestion of the glucose.

The normal fasting glucose in the dog ranges from 70 to 100 mg%. The peak level is seen usually at the one-half hour sample; occasionally it is seen at the one-hour sample. The peak level is usually less than 160 mg%; however, the actual height of this peak is less important than the speed of the animal in returning glucose to the fasting level. The blood glucose should be essentially back to the fasting level within two hours. In many dogs the blood glucose may go slightly below the fasting level before it eventually stabilizes at about the fasting level. This slight hypoglycemic phase usually occurs between the second and fourth hours.

A range of normal values has been reported for all of the different points on the glucose tolerance curve. A fasting blood glucose of greater than 110 mg% is considered abnormal, as is a peak level of greater than 160 mg%. The two-hour level is abnormal if it is elevated above 120 mg%. Some clinicians require that at least two of these values be above normal in order to establish a diagnosis of diabetes mellitus.

Diseases other than diabetes mellitus regularly produce abnormal OGTT curves. Hyperglycemic curves may be seen associated with pheochromocytoma, Cushing's syndrome, acromegaly, and occasionally thyrotoxicosis. In patients with hypothyroidism a flat OGTT curve is usual, due to the decreased intestinal absorption of glucose. Other nonendocrine conditions, such as liver dysfunction and chronic renal disease with azotemia, may also produce abnormal OGTT responses.

Intravenous Glucose Tolerance Test (IVGTT)

The IVGTT was devised to eliminate some of the objections to the OGTT. In particular the intravenous route eliminates any variable due to an absorptive factor's effect on the transport of glucose from the gastrointestinal tract to the bloodstream. Usually ½ g of glucose per pound of body weight is injected intravenously. The calculated dose is administered intravenously using a 50% dextrose solution over a three- to five-minute period. Blood samples are taken at fasting (just before administration of glucose), 15 minutes, one-half, one, two, and four hours after glucose administration. Normally the peak or maximum glucose level occurs after 15 minutes. With progressive samples the level of glucose declines, and the fasting level is reached in approximately one hour.

Interpretation of the IVGTT is similar to that of the OGTT except that the peak is seen earlier, and the return to the fasting or normal glucose level is more rapid. The height of the curve is of minor significance. In the dog with overt diabetes, the blood glucose level is significantly elevated at one hour, and this high level may persist for the four hours. Many of the factors that modify the OGTT may have an identical effect on the IVGTT, except that the IVGTT eliminates any alimentary influences that may occur with the OGTT.

Cortisone Oral Glucose Tolerance Test

This test is occasionally used in man as an attempt to increase the sensitivity of the OGTT. The strength of this technique is that it magnifies slight degrees of defective carbohydrate tolerance and increases the number of abnormal curves in certain patients. Although this procedure is similar to the OGTT, corticosteroids are also administered according to a definite schedule, shortly before the test. This test is primarily a research tool in human medicine, and there are no reports on its use for evaluating spontaneous diabetes in the dog. The usefulness of the cortisone OGTT lies mainly in its ability to detect probable diabetes in persons with minimally decreased carbohydrate tolerance.

Intravenous Tolbutamide Response Test (TRT)

Tolbutamide is a sulfonylurea that stimulates insulin secretion. Although used in man as a test for diabetes, the TRT has no value for diagnosing diabetes in dogs. Most diabetic dogs have an absolute insulin insufficiency and are, therefore, unresponsive to tolbutamide.

The TRT does have value in the dog with certain other abnormalities, especially the suspected insulin-secreting tumor. The standard dose of tolbutamide used in this test in the dog is 10 mg/kg of body weight. Tolbutamide is injected intravenously, and the blood glucose levels are determined as in the OGTT. In the normal dog the blood glucose at one hour decreases to 67.0 ± 1.5% of the fasting level. It continues to drop, and is 64.0 ± 2.2% of the fasting level at two hours. Four hours postinjection the blood glucose level increases to 72.0 ± 1.9% of the fasting level.

Precautions must be taken when utilizing the TRT for the evaluation of an insulin-secreting tumor, since intravenous tolbutamide administration may stimulate the tumor to secrete large amounts of insulin and precipitate convulsions. If convulsions occur, they should be controlled by administering 50% dextrose intravenously to effect.

Radioimmunoassay of Insulin

Quantitation of serum levels of canine insulin have been carried out using a radioimmunoassay procedure. A number of techniques have been described, but most are essentially modifications of a double antibody radioimmunoassay. The basis of the double antibody radioimmunoassay method is to cause insulin to react with anti-insulin antibodies obtained from immunized guinea pigs. The antibody-antigen complex formed is soluble, but can be precipitated by adding anti-guinea-pig globulin antibody obtained from immunized rabbits. When trace amounts of radioactive insulin are added to the serum sample, the amount of native or unlabeled insulin in the sample can be quantitated, since the amount of radioisotope in the precipitate is inversely proportional to the amount of unlabeled insulin in the sample.

Utilizing a double antibody radioimmunoassay procedure following an IVGTT, serum insulin concentrations have been reported in the fasting dog as 20 ± 7 μU/ml, with a range of 9 to 32 μU/ml (Fig. 9–3). Fifteen minutes after administration of glucose, serum insulin concentration increases to 97 ± 43 μU/ml. Thirty minutes later, serum insulin concentrations are 42 ± 24 μU/ml. At one, two, and four hours after the glucose is given, serum insulin concentrations are 17 ± 5, 21 ± 5, and 18 ± 4 μU/ml respectively; these values are not significantly different from concentrations in the dogs during fasting.

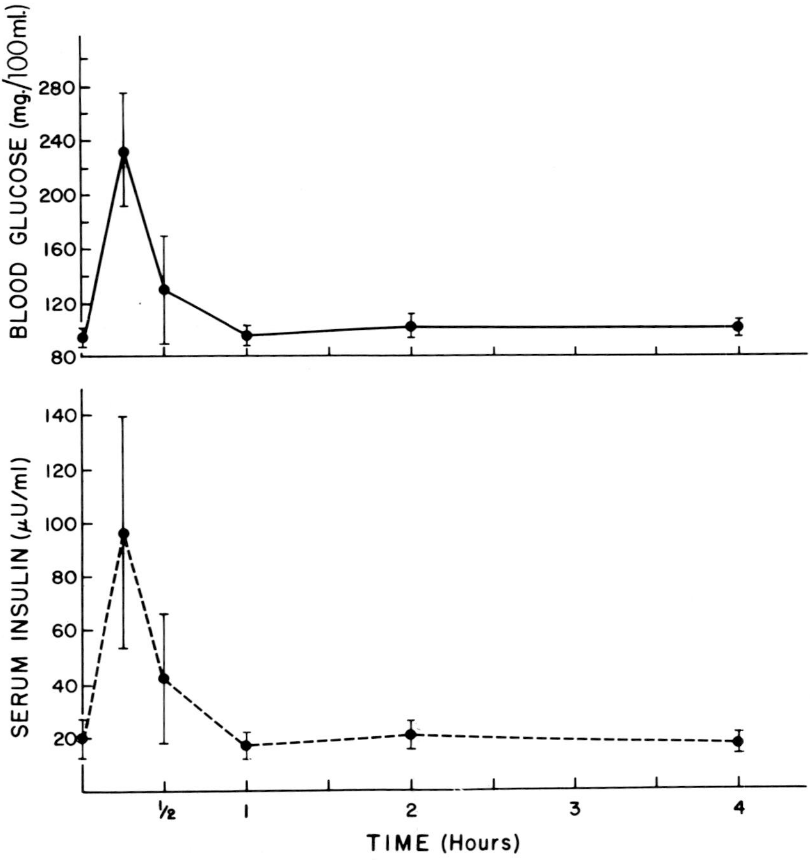

Fig. 9–3. Blood glucose and serum insulin concentrations in seven normal dogs during an intravenous glucose tolerance test. (From Beglinger, R. E., and Siegel, E. T.: Am. J. Vet. Res., *33*:2149, 1972.)

Diagnostic Use of Glucagon

Since glucagon produces hyperglycemia via its potent action on hepatic glycogenolysis, it has been used to study glycogen storage diseases, insulin-secreting tumors, and suspected pheochromocytomas. Glucagon is especially useful in the last situation because it has a direct stimulatory action on the release of catecholamines. This use of glucagon has many advantages over histamine, another drug that is used as a provocative agent in the diagnosis of pheochromocytoma.

Failure of glucagon to produce hyperglycemia connotes defective hepatic glycogenolysis; thus, it is useful in certain glycogen storage diseases. In addition, failure to produce significant or sustained hyperglycemia indicates that the patient has an insulin-secreting tumor. In addition, elevations in serum insulin levels are characteristic of the insulinoma.

Administration of 0.5 mg of glucagon intramuscularly in the normal dog produces an increased blood glucose in about 30 minutes, usually 200% above that of the preinjection level. The blood glucose remains above normal for more than one hour.

Assay of Glucagon

Radioimmunoassay of glucagon has been available since the time when antiserum could be produced for glucagon. However, a number of investigators have reported differences in the specificity of their assay procedures. Essentially two factors interfere with the specificity of the radioimmunoassay procedure of glucagon. One, blood has proteolytic enzymes capable of destroying isotopically labeled glucagon. Recently the addition of proteinase inhibitors appears to protect the radioactive glucagon against these enzymes. There is also more than one material in the blood that is immunologically similar, if not identical, to pancreatic glucagon. Although most of this material is probably gastrointestinal glucagon, even this extrapancreatic glucagon is apparently more than one material.

Present evidence suggests that gastrointestinal glucagon is composed of two fractions of different molecular weights. One of these materials, "true" gastrointestinal glucagon, is biologically, immunologically, and physicochemically identical to pancreatic glucagon. The other fraction, "glucagon-like immunoreactivity," appears to be different biologically from pancreatic glucagon. It is still demonstrable by the radioimmunoassay for glucagon, but this procedure is restricted to specific experimental studies.

Rapid Clinical Tests

Caution must be exercised in the use and interpretation of the rapid techniques for determination of glucose, such as the impregnated cellulose strip (Clinistix). These test strips, which are glucose-specific, have become established as a reliable technique for assessing glucose concentrations in human urine.

However, with experience in the use of these materials with dog urine, there is occasionally poor correlation between significant hyperglycemia and the presence of glucose in the urine. Moreover, some dogs with high blood glucose concentrations show no urinary glucose using the strip test, although glucose can be detected using the less specific tablet test (Clinitest). This latter method detects reducing substances. The cellulose strip test may be unreliable for dog urine due to the high level of ascorbic acid that is excreted into canine urine. It is preferable to use the tablet test for assessing urine concentrations of glucose in the dog, although this technique is not specific for glucose.

The availability of nitroprusside tablets (Acetest Tablets) allows ketone detection in plasma through a simple and rapid test. By implication, the relative degree of acidosis can be estimated (without the need for complicated apparatus) by the degree of ketosis found with the simplified tests using four different concentrations of the serum (undiluted, 50% concentration, 25% concentration, and 12.5% concentration).

Procedure: Place 5 drops of water into three test tubes (Fig. 9–4). The undiluted serum is added to another test tube. From the undiluted serum take 5 drops and add them to one of the tubes containing 5 drops of water. Now there is a 50% concentration in the second tube. Then 5 drops from the second tube are transferred to the third tube, pro-

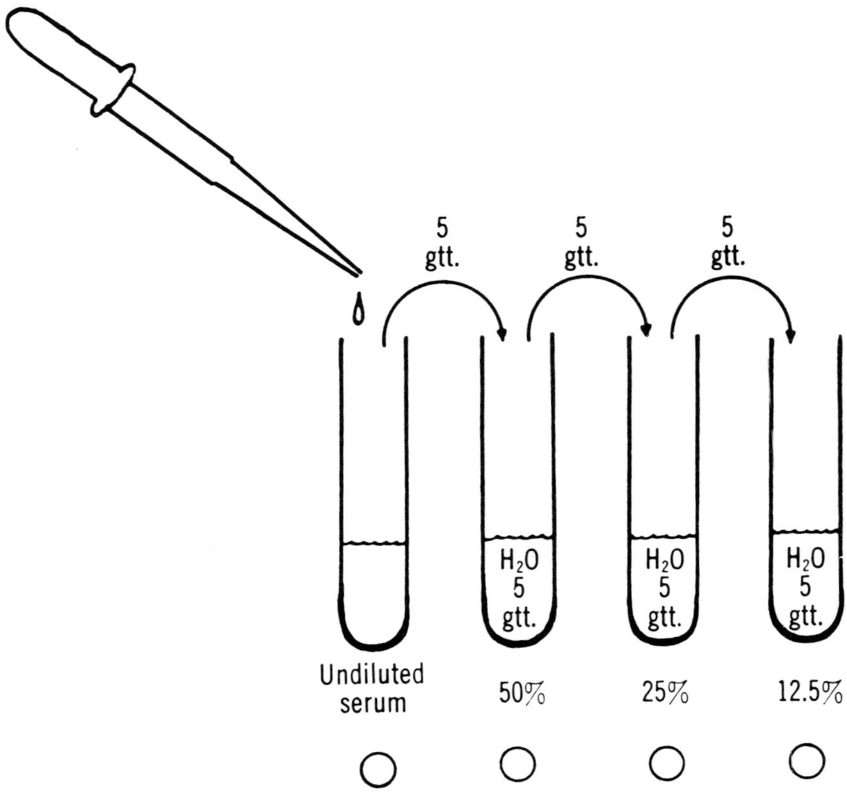

Fig. 9–4. Plasma or serum acetone concentration in dilutions. (From Johnson, R. D.: Postgrad. Med., 39:246, 1966.)

ducing a 25% concentration. Next, 5 drops are taken from the third tube and added to the fourth, resulting in a final concentration of 12.5%. One drop of material from each tube is withdrawn and put on the surface of a nitroprusside tablet. If the tablet becomes purple, the reaction is positive. Since a positive reaction in the very dilute sample signifies a greater degree of ketosis than a reaction in only the undiluted serum, the degree of ketosis can be scored; the undiluted serum is scored +1, increasing through the dilutions until the 12.5% concentration and most dilute sample is scored a +4.

HYPOFUNCTION: DIABETES MELLITUS

The first description in the literature of the association between sugar in the urine and diabetes appeared in 1674 when Thomas Willis wrote "the urine in all whom I have ever met with, . . ., was wonderfully sweet, as if saturated with honey or sugar." In 1815 Chevreul noted that the sweet substance in the urine was identical to grape sugar. However, the importance of the pancreas in the disorder, diabetes mellitus, was not appreciated until 1889 when Minkowski first reported that complete removal of the pancreas in dogs produced diabetes mellitus. Shortly after these experiments, it was suggested that the islets of Langerhans were probably of importance in the pathogenesis of diabetes mellitus.

Finally in 1921 Banting and Best demonstrated that an injection of a pancreatic extract, which they called "insulin," maintained the life of patients with severe diabetes. Thus, they decided that a lack of insulin was the primary pathogenic event in diabetes mellitus. Since the early experiments of Banting and Best, the original theory of an absolute insufficiency of insulin has slowly been eroded; in the last 15 or 20 years abundant new evidence has shed more light and introduced controversy on the true pathogenic and metabolic defect in diabetes.

With the advent of radioimmunoassay techniques to measure insulin, circulating insulin levels were found to be either normal or higher than normal in maturity-onset diabetes in man. This finding has stimulated a continuing dialog on the insulin insufficiency theory. At present two well-defined hypotheses offer an explanation for the etiology of diabetes. In one the proponents suggest that diabetes mellitus results from either an absolute or relative insulin insufficiency. In recent years another group has postulated that either relative or absolute hyperglucagonemia along with insulin abnormalities is important in the development of diabetes. This bihormonal-abnormality theory holds that the major consequences of absolute or relative insulin lack is glucose underutilization, and the absolute or relative glucagon excess is the principal factor in glucose overproduction in the diabetic patient.

Classification

Along with the controversy on the etiology of diabetes mellitus, there is also controversy on the definition and classification of different stages of the disease. Diabetes mellitus is generally accepted to be a disorder of metabolism that, when fully developed clinically, is characterized by fasting hyperglycemia. However, while fasting hyperglycemia is the hallmark of *overt* diabetes, endocrinologists agree that diabetes mellitus can be recognized without fasting hyperglycemia. In man specific vascular and neuropathic abnormalities occur with the disturbance of carbohydrate metabolism.

Since the severity of diabetes can vary and the disorder has an origin and a progression, a number of classification schemes subdivide the disease into certain arbitrary stages. The usual classifications are based on the presence or absence of abnormal carbohydrate metabolism. The earliest state, called *prediabetes*, may progress into *subclinical diabetes;* further progression leads to *latent diabetes;* and the final state is *overt diabetes.*

Prediabetes

The very early stage of "spontaneous" diabetes is termed prediabetes. This stage exists prior to the onset of any specific signs that would identify the disease. The prediabetic individual has a high potentiality for developing diabetes, but none of the usual clinical tests are abnormal. These individuals may be the nondiabetic identical twin of a known diabetic, or the nondiabetic offspring of two diabetic parents. The fasting blood sugar is normal in the prediabetic as is the glucose tolerance test. Some prediabetic people have a slightly decreased or delayed plasma insulin response following a glucose load. However, prediabetes is the stage in which there are genetic grounds to suspect that diabetes may develop, but most of the standard laboratory tests are essentially normal.

Subclinical Diabetes

As prediabetes progresses, the next most easily recognized stage is subclinical diabetes. The fasting blood glucose and the glucose tolerance test are still normal in this stage, but the cortisone-glucose tolerance test is abnormal. These individuals demonstrate some evidence of an insufficient functional reserve of the islet cells. This stage of diabetes often becomes noticeable in pregnant women. They have normal glucose tolerance tests except during pregnancy, at which time the tolerance test becomes definitely abnormal.

Latent Diabetes

This stage immediately precedes overt diabetes. The affected individual does not demonstrate symptoms usually associated with diabetes, but a definite diagnosis of diabetes can be established utilizing routine laboratory procedures. The fasting blood glucose may be normal or elevated, and the glucose tolerance curve is definitely abnormal. The latent diabetic is also termed the chemical or asymptomatic diabetic.

Overt Diabetes

The most advanced stage of diabetes mellitus occurs when there is full clinical expression of the disease. This stage is the most easily recognizable, and classically there is fasting hyperglycemia and glycosuria. Although the glucose tolerance test is abnormal, it is not needed to make a diagnosis. In fact, it is usually not indicated, since the glucose tolerance test may increase the severity of the disease in the overt diabetic.

At present, overt diabetes is readily recognized in veterinary medicine. With more awareness, the earlier stages of the disease will become more recognizable.

Etiology

The etiology is known in only a small percentage of cases of diabetes mellitus. It may result from disease that destroys the pancreas, such as carcinoma or necrotizing pancreatitis. Similarly, a small percentage of cases of diabetes occurs secondary to other diseases, such as acromegaly, Cushing's syndrome, or thyrotoxicosis. This type of diabetes has been called "spontaneous" diabetes, while others have termed it "genetic" diabetes. There continues to be a great deal of controversy over the possible causes of diabetes.

Heredity

For many years a genetic component has been considered important in the development of diabetes mellitus. Even so, there is little agreement on how heredity, precisely, fits into the mechanism or pathogenesis of diabetes mellitus. Within the group of spontaneous diabetics, there is evidence of a relationship between heredity and the development of the disease. In man this correlation is easily recognizable since the aggregation of diabetes has been observed within certain families for many years. Similarly, certain species of animals show a high incidence of diabetes in specific inbred strains. Various strains of mice are highly susceptible to the development of diabetes, as are certain desert rodents, such as the Egyptian sand rat. It has been suggested that certain breeds of dogs are more prone to diabetes than others; however, I have not observed this pattern. Epidemiologic studies have not determined any involvement of a genetic factor in the usual case of spontaneous canine diabetes mellitus.

On occasion, it has been reported that a number of dogs within one family developed diabetes. This clustering of cases of spontaneous diabetes within one canine family is, however, rare. This occurrence suggests only that a small number of canine diabetics do have some genetic factors involved in their disease.

In man, genetic diabetics have been extensively studied, and different modes of genetic transmission have been suggested. Some investigators have hypothesized that a simple autosomal recessive inheritance is involved; and in fact others have suggested that this type of genetic transmission is the only simple mode of inheritance compatible with the information available. However, other investigators have found their data to be incompatible with simple autosomal recessive inheritance. Still others have postulated that diabetes is inherited as a simple autosomal dominant trait with incomplete penetrance. In recent years the important inheritance aspects have been viewed as multifactorial or polygenic; i.e., diabetes results from genes at several loci that act together in a quantitative manner. Other theories on the mode of genetic transmission have been put forth, but it is reasonable to suspect that the wide diversification of theories on the inheritance of diabetes is probably a reflection of the basic lack of understanding of the primary defect involved in diabetes. Once the basic pathogenesis of diabetes is known, the place of inheritance in this disorder will be more easily understood.

Viral Infections

A number of recent studies has stimulated intense interest in the relationship between certain viral infections and the development of diabetes mellitus. In one study from Great Britain, investigators found that insulin-dependent diabetics with a recent onset of the disease possessed higher levels of neutralizing antibodies against coxsackie virus, Group B, type 4, than did normal controls or patients with diabetes of relatively long duration. This evidence is probably the most convincing in terms of a possible association between infection with coxsackie virus and diabetes mellitus. Furthermore, diabetes mellitus occurs in cattle convalescing from foot-and-mouth-disease. This occurrence is of interest, since the virus of foot-and-mouth-disease is a member of the picornavirus group, and thus is biologically similar to the coxsackie virus and another virus (EMC) that causes diabetes in mice.

The EMC or encephalomyocarditis virus was originally isolated in Panama in 1960 from the heart of a pig dying with myocarditis. Most laboratory-adapted strains of EMC virus produce a fatal infection in mice, characterized by myocarditis, progressive paralysis, or encephalitis, or all three. In contrast a specific variant, the M type, is relatively nonpathogenic, particularly in older animals. Mice infected with the M variant of EMC virus develop lesions in the islets of Langerhans and an associated diabetes-mellitus-like disease. The pancreatic lesions associated with this variant strain appear to be fairly well restricted to the islet cells, particularly affecting the beta cells. The acinar cells of the pancreas are not affected by this variant.

The EMC viral infection in mice appears to produce a disease that is similar in many respects to spontaneous diabetes mellitus in man. One major difference is that the widespread vascular lesions, which are so important in diabetes mellitus in man, have not yet been demonstrated with the experimental infectious disease.

Although some studies suggest that certain types of diabetes may be caused by viral infections, it has not been proven that spontaneous diabetes mellitus of man and dog is the result of these kinds of infections. In the event that viruses are found to be involved in the development of spontaneous diabetes, this finding does not necessarily exclude some important contributing factor of inheritance. However, before any definite conclusions can be made between the association of viral infection and clinical diabetes mellitus, more data are definitely necessary.

Diabetes Secondary to Other Endocrine Disorders

If defined as a disorder characterized by fasting hyperglycemia and glycosuria, diabetes mellitus is seen secondarily associated with a number of other endocrinopathies. This definition does not imply that the diabetic condition is identical to spontaneous diabetes mellitus.

Just as a glucose intolerance can appear secondarily or coincidently to the development of another endocrine disorder, there is usually a marked improvement or complete abatement of the glucose intolerance if cure of the primary endocrinopathy occurs. In general, diabetes mellitus occurring secondarily to other endocrinopathies has a moderate clinical course. Although ketoacidosis may develop, it is usually a late finding. The major endocrine diseases that can produce a decreased glucose tolerance and a secondary diabetes are acromegaly, Cushing's syndrome, pheochromocytoma, and thyrotoxicosis. Just as diabetes can occur secondary to other endocrine disorders, some patients develop diabetes mellitus as the primary disease, and at a later time an additional endocrinopathy can complicate this condition.

The dog is susceptible to developing permanent diabetes mellitus after even a short treatment with exogenous growth hormone. Although this susceptibility has been demonstrated experimentally, it seems reasonable that the dog is prone to develop diabetes mellitus secondary to spontaneous acromegaly. Since acromegaly is rare, detailed analysis of the relationship between the two disorders has not been possible.

Growth hormone has multiple effects on many tissues, including some that are similar to those of insulin and some that are opposite. Growth hormone and insulin act together to spare amino acids from gluconeogenesis, to increase amino acid entry into cells, and to increase their incorporation into protein. Growth hormone acts predominantly to promote lipolysis, whereas insulin is strongly antilipolytic and lipogenic. The predominant effects of growth hormone in the acromegalic are (1) the resistance to the glucose lowering effect of insulin, presumably due to inhibition of insulin effects in muscle, and (2) a striking increase in plasma insulin concentration at rest and following glucose. Treatment of acromegaly in man, with a restoration of growth hormone levels to normal, often results in improvement of carbohydrate intolerance.

Excessive glucocorticoid secretion by the adrenal glands results in the disorder called Cushing's syndrome. All clinical findings of Cushing's syndrome essentially relate to the effects of the elevated glucocorticoid concentrations. The glucocorticoids themselves impair glucose tolerance. Plasma insulin levels in the diabetic secondary to Cushing's syndrome are elevated above normal, and an enhanced insulin output is seen following the administration of glucose (see Fig. 9–2).

In the dog with Cushing's syndrome, if hyperglycemia and glycosuria develop, and if Cushing's syndrome is corrected by bilateral adrenalectomy, the diabetes becomes less severe. In most cases, diabetes mellitus is permanent, in that the correction of Cushing's syndrome does not result in complete amelioration of the diabetes.

The clinical symptoms associated with functional pheochromocytomas are the result of increased catecholamine secretion. Catecholamines impair carbohydrate tolerance by inhibition of glucose utilization through stimulation of hepatic and muscle glycogenolysis, hepatic glucose production, and lipolysis with mobilization of free fatty acids. An important action of the catecholamines is their direct inhibition of insulin release from the pancreas. Both epinephrine and norepinephrine cause a prompt rise in blood glucose level coincidently with the fall in plasma insulin level. Although the pheochromocytoma may give rise to a persistent diabetic-like syndrome, more commonly it is paroxysmal in nature. This disappearing and reappearing diabetes appears to be related to the uneven secretion by these tumors.

Similarly, with hyperthyroidism there is interference with normal glucose metabolism. Excessive thyroid hormones increase the rate of nearly all metabolic processes in the body, including the absorption, utilization, and production of glucose. Glucose intolerance associated with hyperthyroidism is usually mild, and in some instances may not even require treatment. Some experiments suggest that the catecholamines play an important role in the glucose intolerance associated with hyperthyroidism.

Diabetes Secondary to Pancreatic Destruction

Glucose intolerance develops if a major part of the pancreas is destroyed, by either massive inflammation or invasion by neoplastic tissue. Destruction of the beta cells in the islets of Langerhans results in an insulin insufficiency and the development of diabetes mellitus. One controversy in veterinary medicine concerns the importance of massive pancreatic destruction in the development of diabetes in the dog. Some reports claim that diabetes in dogs is frequently associated

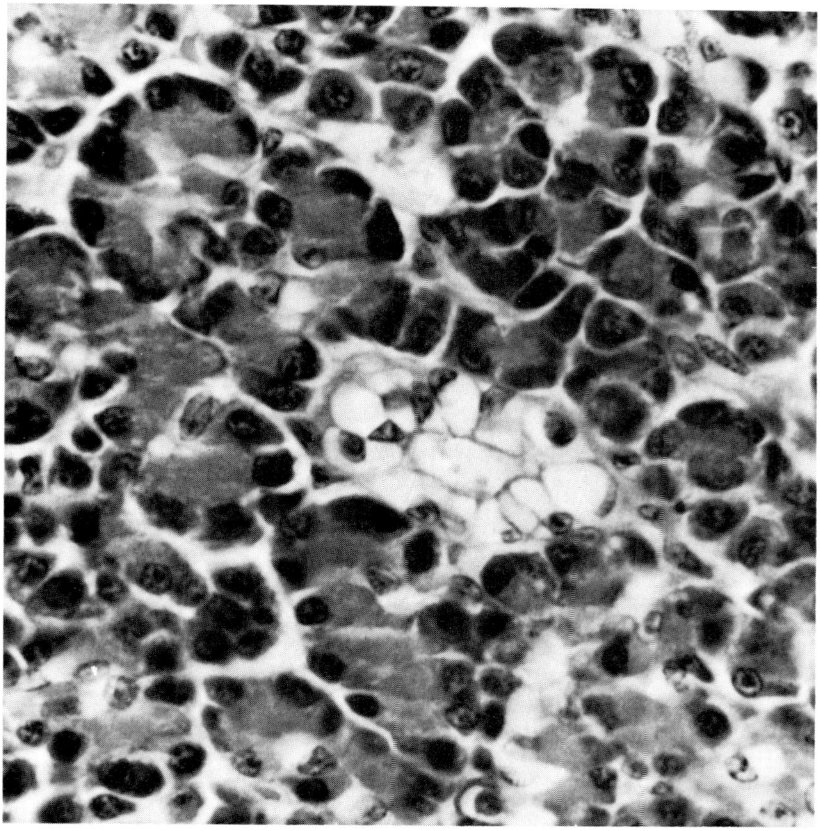

Fig. 9–5. Changes in the islet cells in the dog with spontaneous diabetes mellitus ×408. Hydropic changes (vacuolization) are present in the β-cells. The acinar tissue is unaffected (Courtesy John T. McGrath, University of Pennsylvania.)

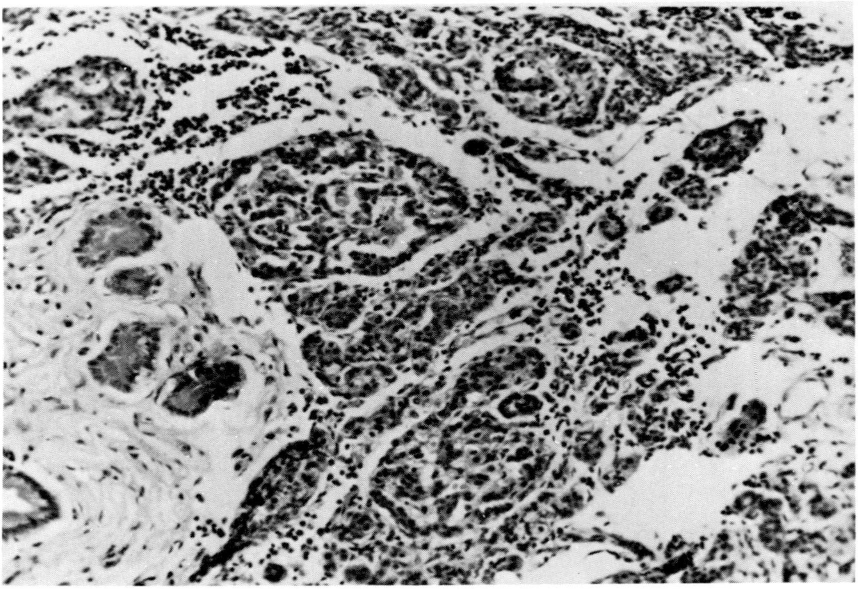

Fig. 9–6. Chronic pancreatitis ×102. There is loss of the normal architecture of the acinar tissue and a sparseness of islets of Langerhans. (Courtesy John T. McGrath, University of Pennsylvania.)

with pancreatitis. Others state that most diabetic dogs do not have destructive changes affecting the acini. The pathologic pancreatic changes in diabetic dogs are primarily seen in the islets of Langerhans (Fig. 9–5).

Some instances of diabetes do occur secondary to pancreatitis (Fig. 9–6). However, most cases of diabetes mellitus that I have seen in the clinic do not have clinical findings supporting the diagnosis of coexisting pancreatitis. Experimentally it has been shown in the dog that, with as little as one-tenth of the pancreas remaining functional, the animal produces enough insulin to prevent the development of diabetes. Therefore, if diabetes develops secondary to destruction of the pancreas, the destruction must be massive, involving at least 90% of the pancreatic tissue.

Pathophysiology

Insulin Insufficiency

Over the years there have been many theories on the primary pathogenic defects of diabetes mellitus. One currently held theory, proposed over 50 years ago, states that an insufficiency of insulin is of predominant importance. The insulin insufficiency may be absolute, as in the juvenile diabetic, or it may be relative in that adequate levels of circulating insulin are not sufficient metabolically. The latter type is seen in man with maturity-onset diabetes in which insulin levels are either normal or slightly elevated. The mechanism for the apparent reduced action of circulating insulin is not established. One theory proposes that antagonistic factors are present in the serum of diabetics. This theory held some favor for a number of years, but has recently been abandoned.

Regardless of the specific defect that results in an insulin insufficiency at the tissue level, those holding the theory of an absolute or relative insulin insufficiency base most, if not all, of the metabolic consequences on this insulinoprivic state. This insulin insufficiency leads to a decrease in the accumulation of body reserve, and an increase in the mobilization of endogenous fuel stores, particularly from mobilization of fat.

In most diabetic dogs, there is an absolute insufficiency of insulin (Fig. 9–7). Insufficient insulin produces a reduced glucose uptake by

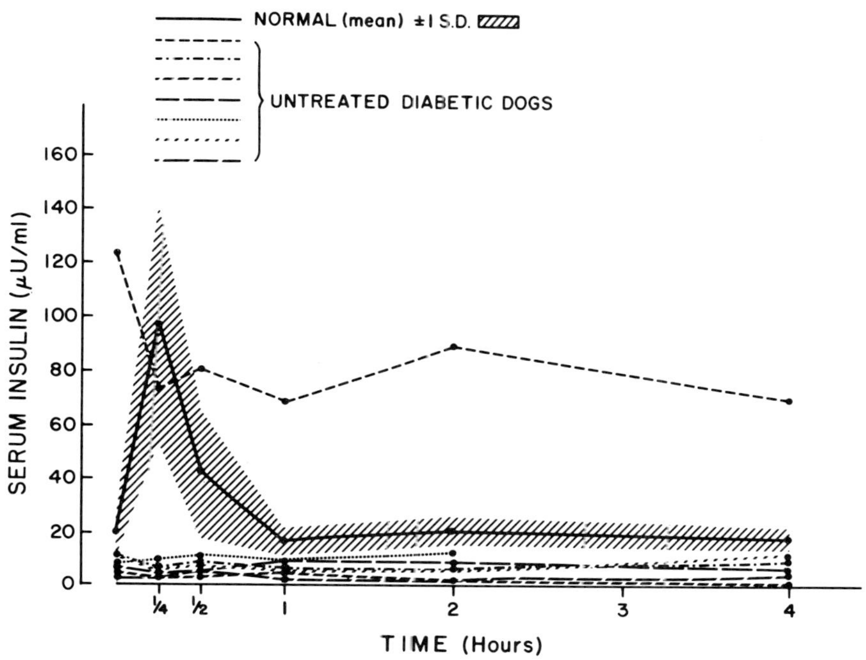

Fig. 9–7. Serum insulin levels in normal and untreated diabetic dogs during an intravenous glucose tolerance test. In six of the seven diabetic dogs the insulin levels were low, and a response was not seen following administration of glucose. One of the seven had higher than normal levels of insulin.

muscle cells and adipose tissue. Amino acids and free fatty acids are increased in circulation. Insulin normally has an inhibitory effect on the breakdown of fats to fatty acids, but in the presence of an insulin insufficiency, lipolysis occurs readily.

The increased free fatty acids are metabolized in the liver to acetyl-CoA. The acetyl-CoA is converted to aceto-acetic acid and beta-hydroxybutyric acid, and in the lung and bladder aceto-acetic acid is converted to acetone. Accumulation of these organic acids produces ketoacidosis. The decreased glucose utilization by peripheral tissues, the increased glycogenolysis, and gluconeogenesis associated with ketoacidosis produce hyperglycemia. As the blood glucose level exceeds the renal threshold (160 to 180 mg% in the dog), glucose is excreted into the urine. Along with glycosuria and obligatory water diuresis, a loss of electrolytes occurs. Excretion of the organic acids, the ketone bodies, results in an increased loss of sodium and potassium. Thus, insulin insufficiency results in hyperglycemia, dehydration with loss of electrolytes, and ketoacidosis.

Insulin Insufficiency/Hyperglucagonemia Hypothesis

According to current studies the metabolic derangements of diabetes mellitus are not completely explained by a simple insulin insufficiency, whether it is relative or absolute. A greater understanding of the physiologic and pathologic actions of glucagon may show that diabetes mellitus is the result of a bihormonal abnormality. Followers of this theory contend that the major consequence of the insulin insufficiency is the glucose underutilization, whereas an absolute or relative hypersecretion of glucagon is an important, if not principal, factor in the overproduction of glucose in the diabetic individual.

Supportive of the bihormonal-abnormality hypothesis is that in all investigated cases, endogenous hyperglycemia was accompanied by relative or absolute hyperglucagonemia. This finding has been shown even after pancreatectomy in the dog. The apparent hypersecretion of glucagon in the pancreatectomized dog certainly is not the result of secretion of pancreatic glucagon. It is extrapancreatic glucagon, believed to be secreted by alpha cells in the gastric fundus and duodenum. These cells are ultrastructurally indistinguishable from the alpha cells in the pancreas. If, however, somatostatin is infused during pancreatectomy and immediately postoperatively, hyperglycemia does not result until the somatostatin infusion is discontinued (Fig. 9–8). Somatostatin is known to have pronounced inhibitory action on both insulin and glucagon secretion. In the pancreatectomized dog hyperglycemia does not result until or in coincidence with the rise in glucagon. Other studies have shown that insulin insufficiency in the absence of glucagon does not result in

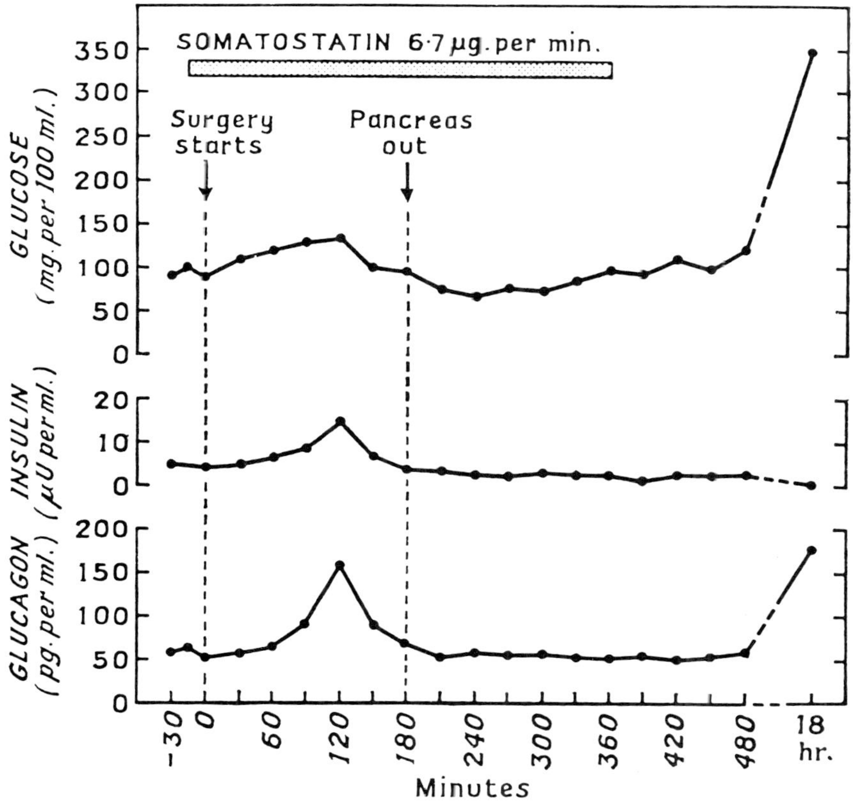

Fig. 9–8. A dog in which somatostatin infusion prevented a rise in plasma glucagon after total pancreatectomy. Despite the absence of measurable plasma insulin, glucose remained below 100 mg/100 ml for five hours after pancreatic resection. Eighteen hours later both glucagon and glucose levels were increased. (From Unger, R. H., and Orci, L. Lancet, *1*:14, 1975.)

hyperglycemia. If glucagon is present, whether administered exogenously or secreted endogenously along with the insulin insufficiency, hyperglycemia quickly results.

A third point in support of this theory is the ability of somatostatin to reduce hyperglycemia in diabetic individuals. This response is related to the glucagon suppressibility of somatostatin. This latter finding offers promise of a new approach to therapy in diabetes.

EARLY CLINICAL SIGNS

With the development of the overt stage of diabetes in the dog, glycosuria appears. This condition produces polyuria and, as a result, polydipsia. Early in the course of the disease, the appetite usually increases; however weight loss appears concurrently. Fasting hyperglycemia is present, and often hepatomegaly is detectable on palpation. In some dogs cataract formation occurs early. If absent when the dog is first examined, the owner should be forewarned about the development of cataracts. Diabetic cataract formation is common in the dog. Most diabetic dogs develop cataracts within six months to a year after the onset of overt diabetes.

LATE CLINICAL SIGNS

With progression of overt diabetes, ketoacidosis and dehydration develop. The clinical signs alter when ketoacidosis is present. In this later stage the animal usually becomes anorexic rather than ravenous for food as he was earlier. Vomiting usually occurs, and diarrhea may be another symptom. The animal becomes more dehydrated and weaker as ketoacidosis progresses. If untreated, the animal may lapse into a diabetic coma.

DIABETIC COMA

Ketoacidotic Coma

The most common cause of coma in the diabetic dog is ketoacidosis resulting from either insufficient treatment with insulin or no treatment. The animal is extremely dehydrated and hypotensive. Respiration is deep and rapid, and because of the severe dehydration and hypotension, urinary output may decrease in the terminal stage.

In a dog presented with diabetic ketoacidosis, abdominal pain may be sufficiently severe to suggest an acute surgical abdomen. Tenderness, abdominal guarding, and decreased bowel sounds may be present without any significant intra-abdominal disease. Often this abdominal tenderness is mistaken for other intra-abdominal disease or for pancreatitis. Although pancreatitis may accompany diabetes mellitus in the dog, the simultaneous occurrence of pancreatitis and diabetes is probably not as common as has been suggested.

Diabetic ketoacidosis can be rapidly confirmed by demonstrating the presence of hyperglycemia and ketonemia utilizing some of the rapid laboratory tests (Dextrostix and Acetest Tablets). Since these methods give only semiquantitative results, it is preferable to measure the degree of ketonemia by diluting the plasma and then quantitating the level of ketones in the different dilutions. However, the nitroprusside reaction (Acetest Tablets) has limitations in that it does not give a positive color change with beta-hydroxybutyric acid. Since it is usually present in plasma at concentrations greater than aceto-acetic acid, significant ketonemia may be present but not demonstrable by this method if the quantities of aceto-acetic acid are not sufficient to give a strongly positive reaction. Fortunately in most clinical situations in which the animal is moderately to severely ketoacidotic, a positive nitroprusside reaction is seen in the undiluted plasma sample. In the diluted samples, however, the concentration of aceto-acetic acid may not be sufficient for an accurate reading.

Since the ketoacidotic diabetic patient is dehydrated, fluids should be administered to expand the intravascular fluid volume. Inadequate hydration is a common and fatal error Isotonic saline solution should be given until adequate hydration is re-established and adequate urinary output is established. If oliguria persists after restoration of normal hydration, coexisting acute renal tubular necrosis may be complicating the ketoacidosis.

After adequate urinary output is established, the water deficit should be corrected since the loss of water usually exceeds that of sodium. Hypotonic solutions, such as one-half strength saline, may be used; however, as time progresses, the potassium deficit must also be corrected. Twenty to 40 mEq of potassium should be administered orally over the first day if the dog is conscious. If the dog is unable to take oral supplementation, potassium can be added directly to the hypotonic saline solution. Certain precautions must be taken whenever potassium is administered intravenously. A rate of 6 to 8 mEq of potassium per hour should not be exceeded without monitoring.

As treatment progresses, the danger of hypokalemia becomes greater. The serum potassium will fall further as renal function improves and as potassium moves into the cell due to insulin therapy. Electrocardiographic monitoring may be useful in detecting either hypokalemia or hyperkalemia; however, this technique is not always sufficiently reliable in determining the level of serum potassium. Since the potassium deficit may be great, it is better to overcompensate with the supplementation if the amount of potassium infused is not greater than 6 to 8 mEq/hour, and provided that urine flow is adequate. A controversial topic is whether bicarbonate should be administered to the ketoacidotic diabetic. In most cases, as fluid and insulin therapy is given, the ketoacidosis abates. However, if severe acidosis is present and the animal is not progressing satisfactorily, 10 to 20 mEq of sodium bicarbonate per 500 ml of one-half strength normal saline solution can be administered.

Another difference of opinion between clinicians concerns the best approach for monitoring the response to insulin therapy in the ketoacidotic diabetic patient. Some clinicians prefer to obtain repeated blood sugar determinations as an index of the success of their therapy. I prefer to monitor blood ketones. The disagreement occurs because blood glucose and plasma ketones do not always decrease in parallel with therapy. I believe that restoration of a nonketotic state is more critical than restoration of a normoglycemic state.

In scoring plasma ketones (as described earlier) when the animal is severely ketoacidotic (plasma ketones, +3 or +4), ½ U of crystalline insulin per pound of body weight is administered subcutaneously, and an identical amount intravenously. Plasma ketones are reassessed in two hours. If plasma ketones remain in the +3 or +4 range, the initial dose of crystalline insulin is repeated. This treatment is continued every two hours until the plasma ketones decrease to the +1 or +2 range. At this time the amount of crystalline insulin is halved by omitting the intravenous dose, and is then administered subcutaneously every two hours until the plasma ketones clear. When a nonketotic state is restored, the dog can be treated with isophane (NPH) insulin.

Lactic Acidotic Coma

In recent years clinicians have recognized that some human diabetics become acidotic, but not ketoacidotic. This acidosis results from an accumulation of lactic acid. The development of lactic acidosis in the diabetic person is usually associated with certain oral hypoglycemic therapy, such as phenformin.

However, since lactic acidosis can develop from hypoxia, hemorrhage, or actual circulatory collapse, it may develop in any diabetic patient, even in those who do not receive phenformin. Whether lactic acidosis occurs in the diabetic dog has not been definitely established, but some clinical evidence shows that it does develop in a small percentage of diabetic dogs. For example, when lactated solutions are the only therapy given to some diabetics, their condition deteriorates. Until this finding is further clarified, it seems judicious not to administer lactated solutions to the moribund diabetic patient. In addition, if lactic acidosis is diagnosed, immediate therapy should be to remove or improve any circulatory collapse or any impediment to tissue oxygenation.

Hyperglycemic-Hyperosmolar Coma

Coma may develop in the nonketotic, nonacidotic diabetic dog. The significant pathologic finding in these individuals is severe hyperglycemia. A blood glucose in excess of 900 mg%, along with dehydration, produces a hyperosmolar-type of coma. Manifestations in this type of coma are hyperglycemia, severe dehydration, hypernatremia, and either stupor or coma. These patients do not show ketosis, and hence have no acetone breath odor. Increase in the hyperosmolar concentration of the serum causes water to be withdrawn from the central nervous system, precipitating the coma.

Therapy should include large amounts of hypotonic solutions, usually 0.45% saline solution intravenously. Usually only small amounts of insulin are necessary in treating this type of diabetes since it is relatively responsive. The fluids should be administered rapidly to reduce the hyperosmolality as soon as possible.

This type of diabetic coma is rare. The response to hypotonic solutions is usually dramatic if administered early in the course of the disease. Only low sodium fluids should be administered because of the hypernatremia present originally.

Hypoglycemic Coma — Insulin Reaction

The most common cause of hypoglycemic coma associated with diabetes mellitus is the excess administration of insulin. Such excesses may result from unnecessarily increased doses of insulin, decreased food intake, or diminished insulin requirements as a result of improved glucose tolerance during exercise. However, less frequently recognized is the association of hypoglycemia with the early development of diabetes, i.e., usually before full clinical manifestations of the diabetic stage are defined.

Although it may seem contradictory that an animal is affected with hypoglycemia in a disease classically characterized by hyperglycemia, this phenomenon results from an abnormal release of insulin by the pancreas. When glucose is taken orally, the normal response is the secretion of insulin by the pancreas. This insulin secretion facilitates the uptake of glucose mainly by muscle and adipose tissue, and it also facilitates the formation of glycogen by the liver. In the early diabetic, insulin secretion may be inadequate or delayed. Therefore, as the blood glucose increases following a normal meal, the balancing or corresponding increase in insulin does not occur to keep the blood glucose within the normal range. The beta cell in the early diabetic has a delayed response, and the insulin peak may occur at a time when the supply of glucose from the intestinal tract is no longer able to buffer its effect. Therefore, the plasma glucose may subsequently fall to hypoglycemic levels. Typically this type of reactive hypoglycemia occurs three to five hours after glucose ingestion.

In the diabetic on treatment, if the hypoglycemic reaction is the result of excessive administration of insulin, the clinical signs are usually seen at a somewhat predictable time after the administration of insulin. The amount of time for the reaction to occur depends on the type of insulin, and corresponds to the time when the insulin is peaking or has its maximum concentration in the circulation. If crystalline insulin is used, the reaction is most commonly seen two to four hours after insulin administration. With NPH insulin, the reaction is more common six to eight hours after administration.

Finally, if protamine zinc insulin is used, the reaction usually occurs somewhere between 14 and 18 hours after insulin administration.

Usually the hypoglycemic coma in the diabetic can be differentiated readily from other diabetic comas. The hypoglycemic coma occurs rapidly and predictably, at a somewhat specific time after the insulin administration. In contrast, ketoacidosis develops over a number of days, during which the animal becomes progressively sicker. Hypoglycemia usually precipitates weakness, incoordination, tachycardia, and/or convulsions. If the hypoglycemia is severe, the animal may lapse into coma showing shallow respirations and severe bradycardia. The hypoglycemic animal is well hydrated, in contrast to the dehydrated state of the ketoacidotic animal.

All of the clinical symptoms of hypoglycemia are rapidly reversed by increasing the plasma glucose. If the animal is slightly incoordinated and is able to eat, a meal is often enough to prevent the hypoglycemic reaction from progressing any further. If, however, the dog is conscious but unable to eat, one should administer a readily available source of glucose per os, for example, honey or karo syrup. In the comatose animal, dextrose is administered intravenously to effect. Occasionally when the hypoglycemic episode is pronounced and lasts any period of time, recovery is slow, and clinical signs appear to be irreversible. In addition, residual cerebral damage may be apparent.

Hypoglycemic reactions can be treated by the owner even if the dog is unconscious. The owner should administer 0.25 to 0.50 mg of glucagon hydrochloride intramuscularly in the unconscious diabetic. This injection usually terminates a hypoglycemic reaction in three to five minutes. After the animal regains consciousness, it should be allowed to eat.

PATHOLOGIC FINDINGS

Pancreatic Lesions

Some reports indicate that inflammatory disease causes widespread destruction of the pancreas in the diabetic dog. This finding is not typical of my experience with spontaneous canine diabetes mellitus. Diabetes does occur secondary to destructive damage of the pancreas (see Fig. 9–6). However, its incidence seems to be overstated in the literature. Inflammatory lesions are seen in the pancreas of some diabetic dogs, but the changes are usually not severe enough to correlate with the severe changes in the islets themselves.

The characteristic finding of spontaneous diabetes in dogs is a reduction in the number and size of the islets, and hydropic degenerative changes in the beta cells (see Fig. 9–5). In cases of diabetic dogs that have been on therapy for long periods of time, the beta cells may disappear completely, leaving behind only residual islets greatly decreased in size, or no islets at all. In many ways the pancreatic lesions in the dog resemble those found in human juvenile diabetics. In some dogs the islet tissue appears quite normal except for some degranulation of the beta cells. This latter change resembles more closely what happens with maturity-onset diabetes in man. This resemblance suggests that at least two major types of diabetes mellitus also occur in the dog. The study of insulin secretions in diabetic dogs seems to confirm this assumption in that most diabetic dogs are absolutely insulin insufficient, similar to juvenile diabetic people, with only a small percentage showing higher insulin levels than normal, more characteristic of maturity-onset diabetes.

Microvascular Lesions

Any modern-day definition of diabetes mellitus in man must include a statement on the carbohydrate intolerance, and must recognize the presence of microangiopathic vascular disease. Based on a strictly morphologic description, the most characteristic change in diabetic microangiopathy is thickening of the capillary basement membrane. Generally, the entire capillary bed of the body is affected, although not uniformly. However, many of the changes reported in different tissues appear to be directly related to the vascularization in that particular tissue. The severe complications in man, diabetic retinopathy and nephropathy, are the result of severe microvascular disease. Over the last half century a great deal of knowledge has been gained concerning treatment of diabetes, but specific understanding of the relationship between the insulin deficient state and the disease of the vascular system remains relatively unknown. Equally important is that, with optimal metabolic control of diabetes, there still appears to be no way to preclude the development of vascular complications.

In the dog, vascular changes somewhat resemble those seen in man. The difference of opinion in the literature seems to relate to the length of time that diabetes has been present in the dog. However, as in man, the longer diabetes is present, the more prevalent the vascular disease.

The changes in the human kidney are rather characteristic in that a specific type of nodular glomerulosclerosis develops. Lesions resembling this type, but not identical, have been found in a small percentage of diabetic dogs. The renal lesions seen in most diabetic dogs are some degree of thickening of the mesangial stalk of the glomerular capillaries, and hypertrophy of the wall of the afferent arterioles.

Peripheral arterial disease is a common complication of human diabetes mellitus. Both large and small vessel lesions may occur, and both may be complicated by pain, neuropathy, and ulceration. This peripheral arterial disease commonly results in such drastic surgical procedures as amputation. In the dog, peripheral vascular disease is not a common complication. It is rare to find peripheral ischemia or gangrene of limbs in the diabetic dog.

Retinopathy

The most common systemic disease causing blindness in man is diabetes mellitus. Whereas such blindness is primarily from diabetic retinopathy, the diabetic dog's blindness commonly results from the development of cataracts.

Diabetic retinopathy is a chronic, progressive disease of the retina, in which microaneurysms usually develop within the vessels of the retina. Small hemorrhages are frequently associated with the microaneurysms. In some an exudative retinopathy may be observed, and these exudates are frequently described as hard or waxy. Other more extensive changes in the retina have been described in man, but controversy has developed over whether typical diabetic retinopathy exists in the dog. The lesions in the retina of the dog seem in many ways similar to those in man. However, failure to find diabetic retinopathy lesions in some dogs is probably related to the length of time that the dog has had diabetes. Similar to man, diabetic retinopathy is usually a rather late clinical development. In the dog with spontaneous diabetes, the retinal vessels show mural pericyte degeneration with "ghost cell" formation. Some microaneurysms are present, usually surrounding zones of focal acellularity. These changes are in many ways indistinguishable from the changes observed in human diabetic retinas.

Pituitary ablation is a rather effective treatment for diabetic retinopathy in man. In a large number of cases, it stabilizes or improves visual acuity. Moreover, the development of angiopathy in the retina is arrested. The mechanism by which pituitary ablation arrests angiopathy and improves vision is unknown.

Cutaneous Changes

Similar to other metabolic disorders, diabetes mellitus may occur in association with cutaneous abnormalities. These cutaneous lesions may be caused by infectious agents, secondary to vascular, metabolic, or nutritional disturbances. Some are idiopathic. For many years it has been reported that diabetic patients are predisposed to cutaneous infections, but this generalization may not be precisely true. Diabetics are not predisposed to develop these lesions; however, when these infections do occur, they are usually more severe and more difficult to bring under control in the diabetic patient. Any type of infection in the diabetic becomes a critical situation since it may cause the diabetes mellitus to get out of control.

Some precise cutaneous lesions in man are seen more frequently in the diabetic than in the nondiabetic. Some of these lesions are the result of specific vascular deficits (necrobiosis lipoidica diabeticorum), or they may be related to increased circulating lipids (eruptive xanthomas). Since the vascular lesions are less severe in the diabetic dog than in the diabetic man, specific canine dermatologic changes associated with vascular disease are not usually seen. In addition, cutaneous lesions associated with hyperlipemia do not appear in the diabetic dog.

Dermatologic changes in the diabetic dog are related somewhat to the state of control of the diabetes. It is more common to find secondary skin lesions in the poorly controlled diabetic dog. If the diabetes is not under adequate control, the animal may have a poor haircoat. Conversely, in the well-controlled diabetic, skin lesions do not appear to be anymore prevalent than in the nondiabetic population.

EFFECT OF ESTROUS CYCLE ON DIABETES

The estrous cycle in the bitch affects diabetes mellitus in a number of ways. Diabetes is more common in the intact bitch than in the spayed bitch or male. The frequency has been reported to be from two to five times more common in the intact female. The higher incidence in the bitch may result from ovarian secretions that accentuate or exaggerate a glucose intolerance. If, as I believe, latent diabetes is more common in the canine population than realized, with ovarian secretions exaggerating glucose intolerance, conversion of latent diabetes into overt diabetes would be expected in the intact bitch.

The clinical signs of diabetes may appear within a few days to a few weeks after estrus. Since the clinical signs of diabetes, such as polydipsia, polyuria, anorexia, vomiting, diarrhea, and dehydration, may be seen as well with pyometra, and since both disorders may be seen shortly after estrus, the two abnormalities may be confused.

The insulin requirements in the treated diabetic fluctuate drastically in most cases throughout the estrous cycle. The insulin requirements begin to increase usually late in proestrus or early estrus, and continue until early metestrus (Fig. 9–9). During metestrus the insulin requirements usually stabilize somewhat, and as the cycle moves into the final stages of metestrus or early anestrus, the insulin requirements drop precipitously. During anestrus much less insulin is required for stabilization.

During pregnancy, insulin requirements increase even more than during the normal nonpregnant cycle (Fig. 9–9). Following parturition the insulin requirements vary depending on whether the puppies are suckling. With suckling, insulin requirements increase, but not to the level during pregnancy. After weaning the insulin requirements

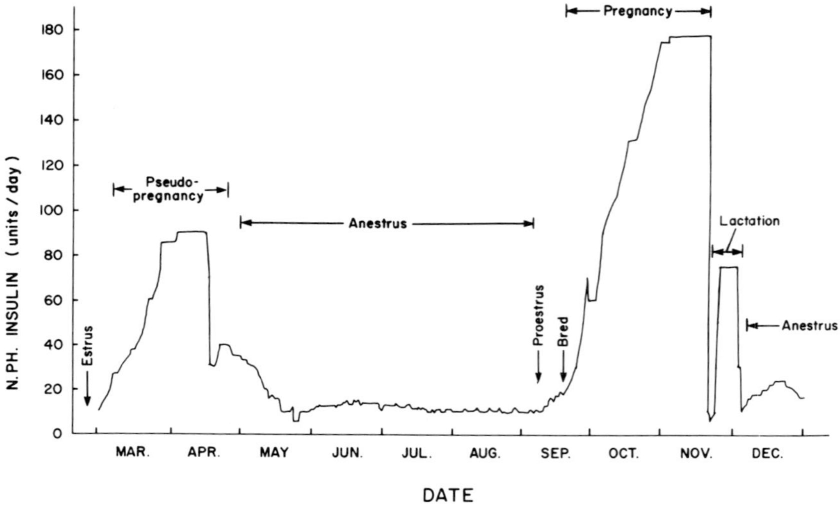

Fig. 9–9. The insulin requirements in a diabetic female dog during the normal estrous cycle and pregnancy. The amount of NPH insulin administered was based on the regimen described on page 129.

decrease quickly to about the level necessary during anestrus. Since the dog does have corpora lutea of lactation, and since insulin requirements during lactation are similar to those during metestrus, it is tempting to infer that the secretion of progesterone, or closely related compounds, is involved in this increased insulin requirement. However, experimental evidence has shown that, while the corpora lutea of metestrus secrete significant amounts of progesterone, the corpora lutea of lactation do not have detectable levels. Thus, while the corpora lutea appear to be related to this increased insulin resistance, the secretion of progesterone is not the only determining factor.

If ovariohysterectomy is performed on a dog that recently was converted into an overt diabetic during or following estrus, complete amelioration of the diabetes may occur. Removal of the ovaries results in reconversion of the overt diabetes to a latent diabetes, and the clinical signs disappear. Thus, spaying of an intact bitch early in the development of diabetes may "cure" the diabetic state. However, more detailed studies would prove that the animal is still a latent diabetic (Fig. 9–10). Since the estrous cycle does have pronounced effects on insulin requirements in the diabetic, I recommend that the bitch be spayed even if the diabetes is permanently overt. This procedure permits a more even control of the diabetes, and the dog requires less insulin.

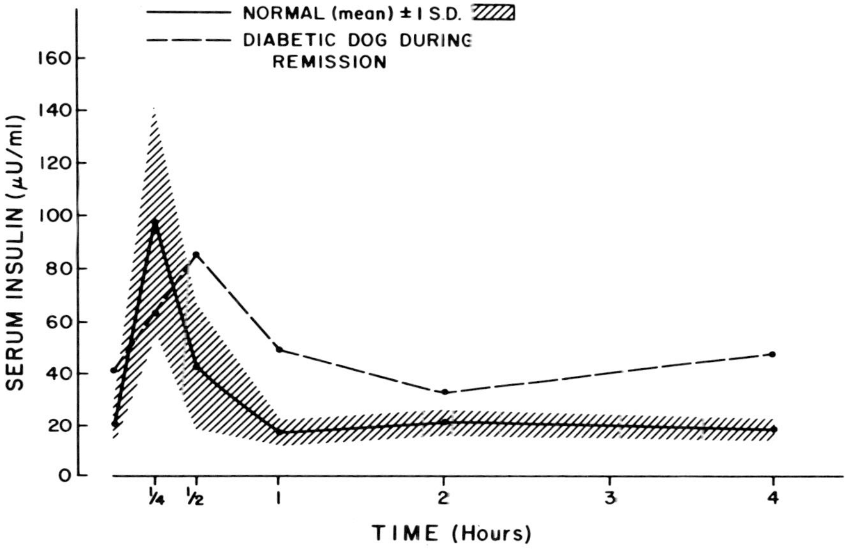

Fig. 9–10. Serum insulin levels in the intact diabetic female bitch during a period of remission (anestrus). The blood glucose levels during the intravenous tolerance test were normal. The insulin levels were higher than normal, and the peak insulin response was slower than normal.

TREATMENT

Diet

It is well established that juvenile diabetes in man cannot be controlled with dietary restrictions alone; chemical control with insulin is also required. In maturity-onset diabetes, some patients may be managed by dietary control alone. Since canine diabetes is usually more closely related to juvenile diabetes, dietary restrictions are not enough to manage the diabetic state. However, in the rare case of canine diabetes resembling maturity-onset human diabetes, control with dietary restrictions alone may be effective. At one time it was recommended that diabetic patients be fed a low carbohydrate, high protein diet. Although this type of diet has been relatively successful, other diets, which differ quite drastically, are also quite successful. Recently a controversy has arisen in human medicine. Since a high protein diet in this country usually also means a high fat diet, and since vascular microangiopathy is an important sequela of human diabetes, some clinicians believe that the high protein/high fat diet is contraindicated in these patients. The opposite, a low carbohydrate diet, may be preferable. Probably the most important aspect of dietary control, at least in the diabetic dog, is that the diet be fairly consistent from one day to another. This regularity produces a more consistent insulin dosage, particularly when exercise is also kept somewhat constant.

In addition to keeping the amount of food constant, it is preferable to divide the amount given over the day into multiple feedings. A major amount of the food should be given one to two hours before the exogenous insulin will be peaking in the bloodstream. When using isophane (NPH) insulin, a preparation that peaks in six to eight hours, one half of the food for the day should be given approximately four hours after the insulin injection.

To balance both the multiple feeding requirement, as well as the larger meal prior to the insulin peak, a system has been established that works relatively well in the dog. One administers isophane (NPH) insulin in the early part of the day, preferably in the morning. One quarter of the daily food is given at the time of the insulin injection. Four hours later, a second, heavier feeding is given. This feeding should contain approximately one half of the food for that day. The remaining one fourth of the food is given during the late afternoon. This type of regime helps to prevent hypoglycemia or insulin reactions.

Insulin Preparations

Various insulin preparations are available. With proper instructions, the owner can control diabetes with various protocols using different insulin preparations.

Crystalline zinc insulin (regular, CZI) has a relatively rapid action. When administered subcutaneously, the peak activity occurs in two to four hours. Total duration of activity usually lasts from five to seven hours in most instances, with a maximum no greater than 12 hours. Because the activity of crystalline insulin is short, it is not usually satisfactory for daily control of diabetes. If it is the only source of insulin, at least two injections are necessary per day. However, crystalline zinc insulin is the insulin to choose when very rapid action is necessary, in particular in the treatment of the ketoacidotic diabetic animal.

Neutral protamine Hagedorn (NPH or isophane) insulin is an intermediate acting insulin. NPH insulin incorporates some of the advantages of CZI, and eliminates some of the disadvantages of protamine zinc insulin. The peak activity of NPH insulin is six to eight hours following subcutaneous administration, and total duration is somewhere between 24 and 26 hours. Because of its duration of effect, it is the preferred insulin for a one-dose-a-day regime.

Protamine zinc insulin (PZI) has prolonged activity — at least 36 hours, with its peak activity occurring 14 to 24 hours after subcutaneous administration. Diabetic dogs that react adversely to NPH insulin, and are not controllable by altering the feeding pattern, can often be controlled with PZI. Since it is active up to 36 hours, a once-a-day regime will produce an additive effect from one day to the next.

Since early 1950 a number of insulins, particularly the lente variations, have been developed. These high-zinc insulin compounds have many characteristics of the other insulins described. *Semilente insulin* is a relatively rapid action insulin, and is in many ways similar to CZI or regular insulin. It has its maximum peak in two to four hours after subcutaneous administration, and has a total duration of approximately 12 to 16 hours.

Lente insulin is an intermediate type of insulin, and is similar to NPH insulin. It has a peak activity in six to twelve hours, with a total duration of 24 to 28 hours.

Ultralente insulin is similar to PZI. It is effective up to 36 hours, with its peak activity occurring 18 to 24 hours after subcutaneous administration.

In addition, mixtures of different insulins are sometimes preferred. Generally, diabetic dogs do best on an intermediate type of insulin, either NPH or lente insulin, for a once-a-day regime. For the ketoacidotic diabetic, crystalline zinc insulin or semilente insulin is preferred for its rapid response.

Ideal Clinical Control

The goal in the treatment of diabetes is to restore, as closely as possible, the normal physiologic relationships. Since insulin secretion normally occurs in response to increasing blood glucose levels, actual physiologic amounts of insulin cannot be administered. In lieu of that solution, the next most sought after situation would be to maintain the diabetic patient as normoglycemic as possible. Theoretically, it would be best if the blood sugar were kept in the normal range throughout the whole day.

For many years the goal in human medicine was to keep the diabetic patient normoglycemic throughout the day in an effort to prevent some of the secondary complications, such as vascular disease. After years of treatment experience, clinicians have fairly well established that, even with the achievement of a fairly constant normoglycemia, no treatment protects a human diabetic against vascular complications.

Diabetic dogs on treatment usually are somewhat more active when they spill small amounts of glucose in the urine. This spillage probably is a reflection of the difficulty of maintaining a constant state of normoglycemia. I suspect that the weakness or lethargy seen in diabetics with frequent negative urine glucose determinations results from a relative hypoglycemia produced during therapy. Recognizing the difficulty in assaying the control of diabetes when the urine glucose is negative makes it easier to stabilize the animal that spills a small amount of glucose in the urine sporadically.

One procedure for controlling nonketotic diabetes in the dog is to initially administer NPH insulin at a dosage of 1 U per 5 pounds of body weight. Each morning the urine is tested for glucose using the Clinitest tablets. If the urine glucose tests +3 or +4, the amount of NPH insulin should be increased by 1 U over the amount given the previous day. However, if the urine glucose is negative or a trace, the amount of insulin is decreased by 1 U. Similarly, if the amount of glucose in the urine is +1 or +2, the amount of NPH insulin administered should be the same as that given the day before. This procedure allows sporadic amounts of glucose in the urine. It does not try to produce normoglycemia, but instead attempts to prevent the development of ketoacidosis.

In addition to measuring urinary glucose, one should also test the urine ketones. Whenever urine ketones are present in the urine for more than one sample throughout a day, or if the level of urinary ketones goes up to moderate or large, the amount of insulin given should be increased from 2 to 5 U per day above that of the day before. This quantity should be continued until the animal again becomes free of ketosis. Ketoacidosis produces a relative insulin resistance, which necessitates the greater amount of insulin.

Increasing the amount of NPH insulin by 1 U per day is preferable in most nonketotic diabetics without complications. However, when large amounts of insulin are needed, as in the intact bitch during estrus or in the diabetic with an infection, the procedure may be too conservative. The mechanism chosen must permit more vigorous treatment when large amounts of insulin are necessary. One method is to have the owner quantitate urinary glucose twice daily (morning and afternoon). If both samples have heavy glucose, that is +3 or +4, on two consecutive days, then double the increase of insulin to 2 U over that of the day before. If after two more days the amount of glucose still remains high in both samples on both days, the amount of insulin should again be doubled, giving now 4 U of insulin above the prior day's administration. By continuing this method, in only a few days insulin levels would be increasing by 16 or 32 U per day. When urinary glucose becomes negative, the amount of insulin can decrease to that of the day before, when the animal was still spilling glucose into the urine. When the glucose is positive in the urine at this level, one can increase the amount of insulin slowly from that point until stabilization occurs.

Insulin Resistance

The insulin resistant individual requires large amounts of insulin for adequate control of diabetes. Since pancreatectomized dogs require 10 to 20 U of insulin per day, any dog needing more than 20 U per day has some type of insulin resistance.

Two major mechanisms result in the development of insulin resistance. The first, an immune response, occurs in some individuals that are able to produce antibodies against the insulin being administered exogenously. This type of insulin resistance has been demonstrated occasionally in man, but it is rare. Insulin antibodies have been demonstrated in many diabetic people on therapy, but generally the antibodies are not neutralizing in action. I do not believe that neutralizing antibody against insulin is a factor of insulin resistance in most diabetic dogs.

Insulin resistance in the dog is mainly the nonimmune type. The most important cause of nonimmune insulin resistance is the development of ketoacidosis. The amount of insulin necessary for control increases greatly in the ketotic animal. In addition, the estrous cycle and probably some sex steroids increase insulin requirements. Ketoacidosis and estrus account for most of the instances of insulin resistance in the dog. Another nonimmune cause is the development of an infection. In many diabetic animals, the development of infection signals the need for greater amounts of insulin.

A less frequent cause of insulin resistance is the development of other endocrinopathies, or the administration of certain drugs. Acromegaly, hyperthyroidism, and Cushing's syndrome foster increased insulin requirements. The administration of growth hormone, thyroxine, or glucocorticoids has an identical effect.

Complications of Insulin Therapy

The greatest difficulty associated with insulin therapy is hypoglycemia, due to excess insulin administration. Since the amount of insulin must be balanced with the amount of exercise and food intake, a hypoglycemic reaction may result if the amount of food is decreased or exercise increased. Insulin allergy or insulin lipodystrophy is rarely seen. With insulin allergy there is a local reaction at the site of injection. The spot is usually red, swollen, and hot, and a subcutaneous nodule may form. This condition usually occurs during the first weeks of therapy, and usually disappears later. The true anaphylactoid type of allergy to insulin is very rare, but urticaria and shock are always a possibility. The other complication associated with the site of injection is lipodystrophy, which may be either lipoatrophy or lipohypertrophy, harmless changes in the subcutaneous fat. In the case of atrophy, the condition involves a sharply delineated loss of fat. With lipohypertrophy the mass produced is composed of fibrous tissue and is relatively avascular. These changes usually occur after repeated doses of insulin administration at the same site. To prevent lipodystrophies, the injection sites should be rotated.

Oral Hypoglycemic Compounds

Of the numerous oral hypoglycemic drugs used to treat diabetes, there are two major types, the sulfonylurea compounds, such as tolbutamide and chlorpropamide, and the biguanide compounds, of which phenformin is representative (Fig. 9–11).

The sulfonylurea compounds are effective mainly because they increase the release of insulin from the beta cells of the islets of Langerhans. Thus, they are useful in treating diabetics that have a responsive pancreas. The compounds are used in man only in maturity-onset diabetes, since insulin levels are relatively high or normal and increase with the use of these compounds. In the diabetic dog, insulin levels are usually absent, which is more typical of juvenile diabetics; thus, the sulfonylurea compounds are not effective therapy. The pancreas of the diabetic dog is not responsive to these drugs. In addition, chronic administration of tolbutamide is hepatotoxic in dogs.

Of the biguanide compounds, phenformin is the only one in general use. Despite considerable investigation, however, its mode of action is not completely understood. Unlike the sulfonylurea preparations, phenformin does not stimulate an increased output of insulin. Present evidence suggests that phenformin has a peripheral effect on insulin action. Phenformin will not lower the blood sugar in the normal dog or the normal person. Its hypoglycemic or glucose-lowering effect is

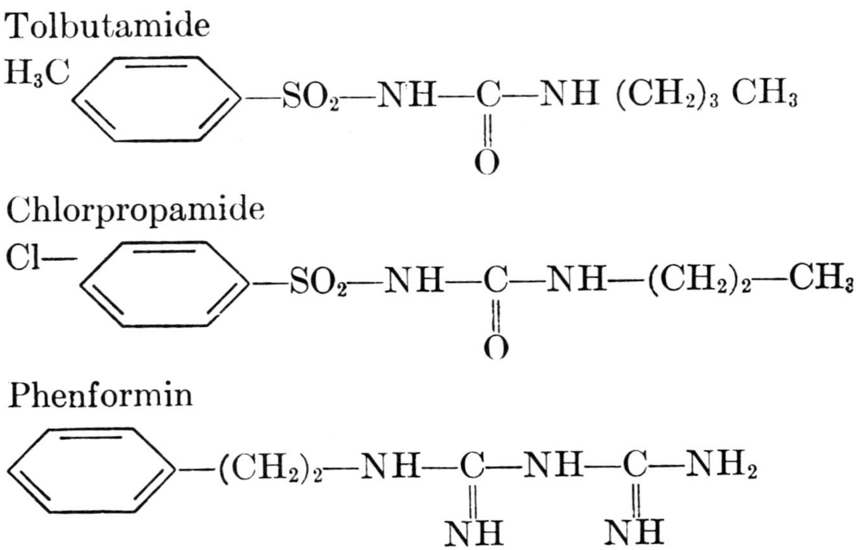

Fig. 9–11. Chemical structure of three commercially available oral hypoglycemic compounds. (From Tomhave, W. G.: Med. Clin. North Am., *47*:53, 1963.)

seen only in the maturity-onset type of diabetes, in which serum insulin levels are present. Since most cases of canine diabetes show an absolute insufficiency of insulin, phenformin would not be effective. The hypoglycemic drugs would be effective only in those rare cases when canine diabetes is accompanied by high serum insulin levels.

A recent controversy concerns whether human diabetics in long-term treatment with oral hypoglycemic drugs have a greater incidence of cardiovascular disease. Whatever the outcome, caution should be exercised when using these drugs in human medicine.

HYPERFUNCTION

A fall in the plasma glucose to a level of 40 mg/100 ml or less may elicit a variety of clinical signs depending on the nature of the stimulus responsible for the fall in plasma glucose, the rate at which the hypoglycemia develops, and the competence of the several contraregulatory mechanisms that normally stabilize the blood glucose.

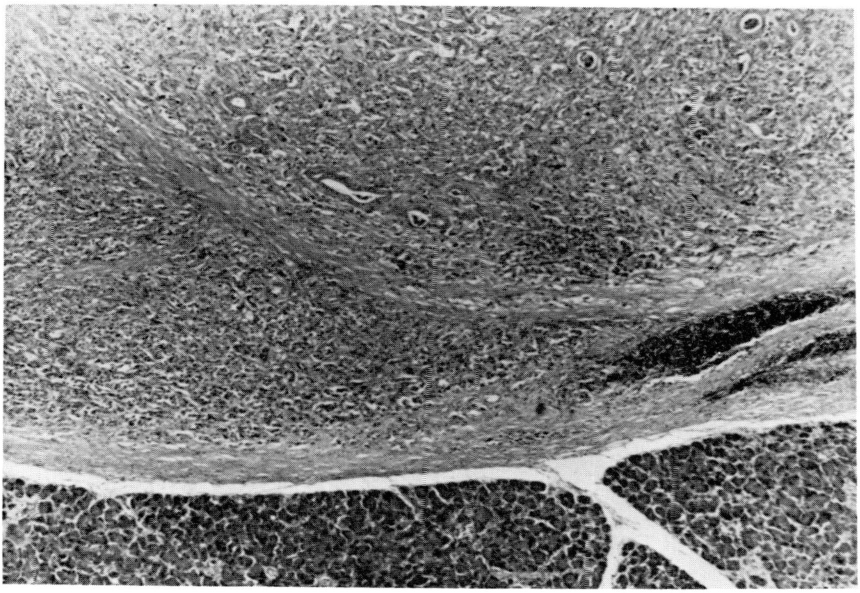

Fig. 9–12. Pancreatic islet-cell adenoma ×34. Normal acinar tissue is seen below, with the islet-cell adenoma being above. The solid pattern of islet-cell tumor is characterized by broad sheets of cells separated by bands of connective tissue hyalin. (Courtesy John T. McGrath, University of Pennsylvania.)

Hypoglycemia does not manifest itself in the same manner in all patients; the symptoms depend mostly upon the duration of the hypoglycemia, and the rate of fall of the blood sugar rather than the final level that it reaches. A rapid decline in blood glucose stimulates a compensatory epinephrine secretion with symptoms related to the autonomic nervous system, such as weakness, hunger, tachycardia, and occasionally trembling. If the blood sugar decreases more slowly and over a prolonged period, frequently the symptoms are more of the central nervous system type, i.e., mental confusion, incoordination, convulsions, and/or coma.

Among the different causes of hypoglycemia, some conditions are organic, in that specific pathologic lesions are associated with the development of hypoglycemia. This category includes hyperinsulinism associated with pancreatic islet-cell tumors, either adenomas or adenocarcinomas (Figs. 9–12 and 9–13). Other organic causes of hypoglycemia in man are pituitary insufficiency, adrenal insufficiency, hepatic dysfunction, and thyroid insufficiency. In the dog these disorders are rarely the cause of hypoglycemia; only with adrenal insufficiency does hypoglycemia develop, and then only terminally.

Numerous instances appear to be functional hyperinsulinism, i.e., a hypersecretion of insulin under certain unusual physiologic stimuli.

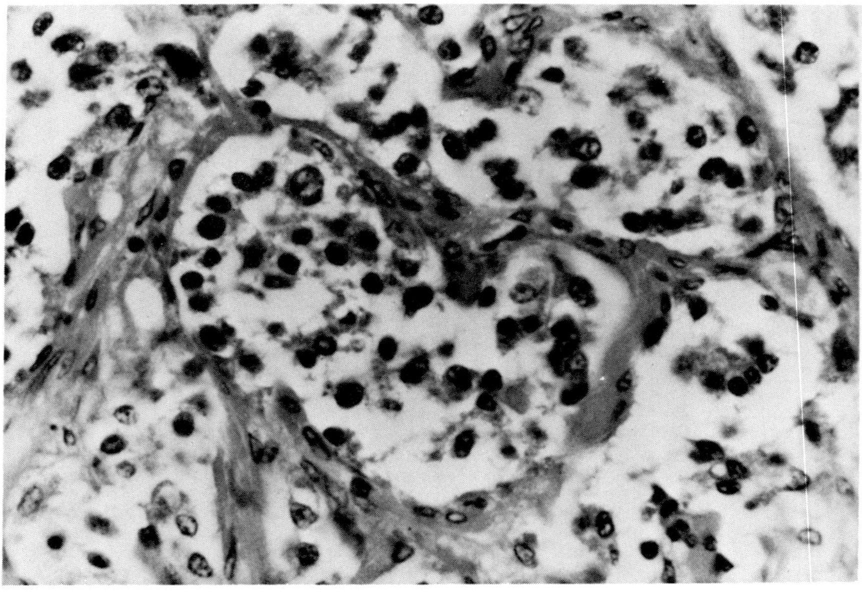

Fig. 9–13. Pancreatic islet-cell adenoma ×289. Higher magnification of Fig. 9–12. The cells of this type of adenoma possess pleomorphic and hyperchromatic nuclei in scant cytoplasm.

When this disorder is present, it is usually seen three to five hours following feeding. The ingestion of a meal containing glucose appears to result in a hypersecretion of insulin and a resulting hypoglycemia. Similarly, hypoglycemia seen in the working breeds of dogs during excessive muscular work appears to be a functional disorder. This type of hypoglycemia can be controlled by altering the diet to provide an even distribution of energy supply over the day.

Various other disorders producing hypoglycemia have been described in man, but most of them have not been studied in any detail in the dog. Leucine sensitivity is seen in certain individuals, who overrespond to leucine ingestion with a hypersecretion of insulin and hypoglycemia. In addition, a number of glycogen storage diseases can produce hypoglycemia. Although glycogen storage diseases probably do exist in the dog, little study has been devoted to the specific biochemical defects associated with these disorders.

HYPERINSULINISM

The most common cause of hypoglycemia in the dog is organic hyperinsulinism, associated with insulin-secreting tumors of the beta cells of the islets of Langerhans. This disease is primarily seen in the dog above five years of age. Although hyperinsulinism has been reported in man associated with only hyperplasia of the beta cells, this disease has not been described in the dog.

Diagnosis of organic hyperinsulinism is based on the presence of Whipple's triad: (1) there is a hypoglycemic attack, which can be precipitated by fasting; (2) during an attack, the blood sugar level is 50 mg% or less; and (3) the symptoms can be relieved promptly by administering glucose orally or intravenously. The fasting blood sugar, when estimated after an overnight fast, may be within normal limits, and the condition may not be accompanied by symptoms. However, if a provocative 24- to 48-hour fast is used, the characteristic hypoglycemia will be evident.

If an intravenous glucose tolerance test is used, the shape of the curve may suggest the presence of hyperinsulinism. Usually if the intravenous tolerance test is diagnostic, the preinjection level is below normal. One hour after injection of the glucose, the blood sugar level frequently returns to the hypoglycemic range. Often prolonged hypoglycemia occurs; i.e., the blood sugar level remains below normal even four hours postinjection. Some reports suggest that glucose tolerance tests are not completely reliable for the diagnosis of insulin-secreting tumors. This has not been my experience.

One procedure that may be helpful for confirming a diagnosis of hyperinsulinism is the intravenous tolbutamide response test. Tolbutamide stimulates an increased secretion of insulin from the normal pancreas and also the β-cell pancreatic tumor. One hour after tolbutamide is injected intravenously into normal dogs (10 mg/kg), the blood sugar decreases to 67 ± 1.5% of the control value. If an insulin-secreting tumor is present, the degree of hypoglycemia is usually more pronounced. It is not unusual to precipitate a hypoglycemic convulsion during the infusion of tolbutamide. Whenever this test is utilized in the insulin-secreting tumor suspect, the veterinarian must be prepared to abort the study with the infusion of dextrose if a hypoglycemic reaction occurs. The degree and persistence of the hypoglycemia induced by tolbutamide are more severe in patients with insulin-secreting tumors than they are in the healthy dog.

With the availability of immunoassay of insulin in canine blood, the diagnosis of hyperinsulinism has become more accurate. Insulin levels should be determined following an intravenous glucose tolerance test, or following the intravenous tolbutamide response test. In most instances the diagnosis of insulin-secreting tumors is relatively straightforward using immunoassay of insulin. Since insulin secretions fluctuate in dogs, the diagnosis should not be based on a single fasting insulin level.

Approximately 60% of the insulin-secreting tumors in dogs originate in the right or duodenal lobe of the pancreas; the remaining 40% are found in the left pancreatic lobe. The tumors may be quite small and difficult to locate during surgery. If a tumor is not found after a positive diagnosis through immunoassay procedures, the preferred procedure is to remove the right lobe of the pancreas.

Many of these insulin-secreting tumors are malignant. Even if they are removed when clinical signs are first seen, the high incidence of metastasis makes the prognosis poor. If evidence of metastasis is not seen at surgery, metastatic lesions may still appear and become functional for up to 1½ years after the original surgery. Recurrence of hypoglycemia following surgery suggests the presence of metastatic lesions. The sites usually affected are the regional lymph nodes and the liver.

Organic hyperinsulinism associated with a pancreatic tumor is not usually difficult to diagnose. First, a complex of clinical signs, called Whipple's triad, usually appears. Absolute confirmation requires serum insulin assay. The treatment of choice is early exploration of the abdomen with removal of the tumor. However, if a tumor is not found after careful palpation of the entire pancreas, resection of that part of the pancreas more commonly affected, that is, the duodenal lobe, is a justifiable procedure.

SELECTED READING

1. Acosta, J. M., et al.: Distribution and volume of the islets of Langerhans in the canine pancreas. Acta Physiol. Latin. Am., *19*:175, 1969.

2. Alberti, K. G. M. M., et al.: Inhibition of insulin secretion by somatostatin. Lancet, *2*:1299, 1973.
3. Alberti, K. G. M. M., Hockaday, T. D. R., and Turner, R. C.: Small doses of intramuscular insulin in the treatment of diabetic coma. Lancet, *2*:515, 1973.
4. Alberti, K. G. M. M., and Hockaday, T. D. R.: Rapid blood ketone body estimation in the diagnosis of diabetic ketoacidosis. Br. Med. J., *2*:565, 1972.
5. Albrink, M. J.: Dietary and drug treatment of hyperlipidemia in diabetes. Diabetes, *23*:913, 1974.
6. Albrink, M. J., and Davidson, P. C.: Dietary therapy and prophylaxis of vascular disease in diabetics. Med. Clin. North Am., *55*:877, 1971.
7. Allen, G. E.: Diabetes mellitus and the skin. Practitioner, *203*:189, 1969.
8. Anderson, N. V., and Johnson, K. H.: Pancreatic carcinoma in the dog. J. Am. Vet. Med. Assoc., *150*:286, 1967.
9. Andres, R.: Aging and diabetes. Med. Clin. North Am., *55*:835, 1971.
10. Arky, R. A., and Arons, D. L.: Hypoglycemia in diabetes mellitus. Med. Clin. North Am., *55*:919, 1971.
11. Arnould, Y., Ooms, H. A., and Franckson, J. R. M.: Analysis of urinary excretion of insulin in the normal dog. Arch. Int. Pharmacodyn. Ther., *167*:480, 1967.
12. Bacon, G. E., and Parkhurst, R. D.: Metabolic considerations in the treatment of juvenile diabetes mellitus. Med. Clin. North Am., *53*:1367, 1969.
13. Balodimos, M. C.: Treatment of diabetic retinopathy. Med. Clin. North Am., *55*:989, 1971.
14. Barker, W. F.: Peripheral vascular disease in diabetes. Med. Clin. North Am., *55*:1045, 1971
15. Beck, A. M., and Krook, L.: Canine insuloma. Two surgical cases with relapses. Cornell Vet., *55*:330, 1965.
16. Beglinger, R. E., and Siegel, E. T.: Double antibody radioimmunoassay in canine serum. Am. J. Vet. Res., *33*:2149, 1972.
17. Belmonte, M. M., Sarkozy, E., and Harpur, E. R.: Urine sugar determination by the two-drop Clinitest method. Diabetes, *16*:557, 1967.
18. Berkow, J. W., and Ricketts, R. L.: Spontaneous diabetes mellitus in dogs. J. Am. Vet. Med. Assoc., *146*:1101, 1965.
19. Bloodworth, J. M. B., Jr., Engerman, R. L., and Powers, K. L.: Experimental diabetic microangiopathy. Diabetes, *18*:455, 1969.
20. Booth, M., and El Garf, T. A. R.: Plasma progesterone concentration during the third trimester of diabetic pregnancy. J. Obstet. Gynaecol. Br. Commonw., *81*:768, 1974.
21. Braverman, I. M.: Cutaneous manifestations of diabetes mellitus. Med. Clin. North Am., *55*:1019, 1971.
22. Bressler, R., and Galloway, J. A.: Insulin treatment of diabetes mellitus. Med. Clin. North Am., *55*:861, 1971.
23. Campbell, J., and Rastogi, K. S.: Effects of glucagon and epinephrine on serum insulin and insulin secretion in dogs. Endocrinology, *79*:830, 1966.
24. Capen, C. C., and Martin, S. L.: Hyperinsulinism in dogs with neoplasia of the pancreatic islets. Vet. Pathol., *6*:309, 1969.
25. Cole, H. S., and Camerini-Davalos, R. A.: Diet therapy of diabetes mellitus. Med. Clin. North Am., *54*:1577, 1970.
26. Coleman, T. J., Taylor, K. W., and Gamble, D. R.: The development of diabetes following coxsackie B virus infection in mice. Diabetologia, *10*:755, 1974.
27. Colwell, A. R., Jr., and Zuckerman, L.: Regulation of insulin release by pancreatic glucagon. Diabetes, *19*:429, 1970.
28. Cotton, R. B., Cornelius, L. M., and Theran, P.: Diabetes mellitus in the dog: a clinicopathologic study. J. Am. Vet. Med. Assoc., *159*:863, 1971.
29. Danowski, T. S.: Non-ketotic coma and diabetes mellitus. Med. Clin. North Am., *55*:913, 1971.
30. Dube, A. H.: Diabetes teaching manual for patients and hospital personnel. N. Y. State J. Med., *69*:1169, 1969.
31. Duckworth, W. C., and Kitabchi, A. E.: Direct measurement of plasma proinsulin in normal and diabetic subjects. Am. J. Med., *53*:418, 1972.

32. Dundon, S., Murphy, A., and Raftery, J.: Diabetes mellitus in childhood. J. Ir. Med. Assoc., *67*:503, 1974.
33. Eliasson, S. G.: Disorders of the nervous system in diabetes. Med. Clin. North Am., *55*:1001, 1971.
34. Emmer, M., Gorden, P., and Roth, J.: Diabetes in association with other endocrine disorders. Med. Clin. North Am., *55*:1057, 1971.
35. Etheridge, J. E., Jr.: Hypoglycemia and the central nervous system. Pediatr. Clin. North Am., *14*:865, 1967.
36. Fajans, S. S.: What is diabetes? Med. Clin. North Am., *55*:793, 1971.
37. Felig, P.: Pathophysiology of diabetes mellitus. Med. Clin. North Am., *55*:821, 1971.
38. Fischer, U., et al.: Insulin and insulin effect in a she-dog with spontaneous diabetes. Horm. Metab. Res., *2*:251, 1970.
39. Foa, P. P.: Glucagon: An incomplete and biased review with selected references. Am. Zool., *13*:613, 1973.
40. Frawley, T. F., and Pensuwan, S.: Hypoglycemia: tolbutamide and leucine tests in insulinoma. Med. Clin. North Am., *52*:283, 1968.
41. Gamble, D. R.: Epidemiological and virological observations on juvenile diabetes. Postgrad. Med. J., *50* (Suppl. 3):528, 1974.
42. Gepts, W., and Toussaint, D.: Spontaneous diabetes in dogs and cats. Diabetologia, *3*:249, 1967.
43. Gerich, J. E., et al.: Prevention of human diabetic ketoacidosis by somatostatin. N. Engl. J. Med., *292*:985, 1975.
44. Gerich, J. E., et al.: Inhibition of pancreatic glucagon responses to arginine by somatostatin in normal man and in insulin-dependent diabetics. Diabetes, *23*:876, 1974.
45. Gerich, J. E., et al.: Effect of somatostatin on plasma glucose and insulin responses to glucagon and tolbutamide in man. J. Clin. Endocrinol. Metab., *39*:1057, 1974.
46. Glick, G.: Glucagon. Circulation, *45*:513, 1972.
47. Goetz, F. C.: Management of adult-onset diabetes. Postgrad. Med., *52*:63, 1972.
48. Goldberg, M. F.: Natural history of diabetic retinopathy. Isr. J. Med. Sci., *8*:1311, 1972.
49. Gordon, E. S.: Diabetes mellitus: new developments. Postgrad. Med., *55*:145, 1974.
50. Grillo, T. A. I., and Cunningham, J. G.: Serum insulin in totally pancreatectomized pregnant dogs. J. Endocrinol., *39*:307, 1967.
51. Hausler, H. R., Sibay, T. M., and Campbell, J.: Retinopathy in a dog following diabetes induced by growth hormone. Diabetes, *13*:122, 1964.
52. Hellerstrom, C., et al.: Aspects of the biosynthesis of glucagon in mammals. Postgrad. Med. J. (August Suppl.), *49*:601, 1973.
53. Hellman, B., Wallgren, A., and Hellerstrom, C.: Two types of islet α cells in different parts of the pancreas of the dog. Nature, *194*:1201, 1962.
54. Hommel, H., Fischer, U., and Kansy, H.: Insulin in the pancreatic blood and insulin half-life in an Alsatian bitch with spontaneous diabetes. Horm. Metab. Res., *3*:213, 1971.
55. Horger, E. O., III, Miller, M. C., III, and Conner, E. D.: Relation of large birthweight to maternal diabetes mellitus. Obstet. Gynecol., *45*:150, 1975.
56. Horger, E. O., III, Kellett, W. W., and Williamson, H. O.: Diabetes in pregnancy. Obstet. Gynecol., *30*:46, 1967.
57. Idezuki, Y., et al.: Experimental pancreaticoduodenal preservation and transplantation. Surg. Gynecol. Obstet., *126*:1002, 1968.
58. Johnson, R. D.: Management of diabetic keotacidosis. Postgrad. Med., *39*:246, 1966.
59. Kahil, M. E., et al.: Alcohol and the tolbutamide response in the dog. J. Lab. Clin. Med., *64*:808, 1964.
60. Kemp, C. B., et al.: Effect of transplantation site on the results of pancreatic islet isografts in diabetic rats. Diabetologia, *9*:486, 1973.
61. Ketterer, H., Eisentraut, A. M., and Unger, R. H.: Effect upon insulin secretion of physiologic doses of glucagon administered via the portal vein. Diabetes, *16*:283, 1967.

62. King, J. M., Kavanaugh, J. F., and Bentinck-Smith, J.: Diabetes mellitus with pituitary neoplasms in a horse and a dog. Cornell Vet., *52*:133, 1962.
63. Knisley, R. E., and Marsh, F. G.: Lipotrophic diabetes. South Med J., *62*:514, 1969.
64. Koerker, D. J., et al.: Somatostatin: hypothalamic inhibitor of the endocrine pancreas. Science, *184*:482, 1974.
65. Kolodny, R. C., et al.: Sexual dysfunction in diabetic men. Diabetes, *23*:306, 1974.
66. Koutras, P., and White, R. R.: Insulin-secreting tumors of the pancreas. Surg. Clin. North Am., *52*:299, 1972.
67. Krahl, M. E.: Endocrine function of the pancreas. Annu. Rev. Physiol., *36*:331, 1974.
68. Kramp, R. C., Congdon, C. C., and Smith, L. H.: Recovery from experimental diabetes mellitus in mice after pancreas transplantation. Diabetes, *23*:183, 1974.
69. Kreisberg, R. A., et al.: Insulin secretion in obesity. N. Engl. J. Med., *276*:314, 1967.
70. Kumar, D., Mehtalia, S. D., and Miller, L. V.: Diagnostic use of glucagon-induced insulin response. Ann. Intern. Med., *80*:697, 1974.
71. Kuzuya, T., Kajinuma, H., and Ide, T.: Effect of intrapancreatic injection of potassium and calcium on insulin and glucagon secretion in dogs. Diabetes, *23*:55, 1974.
72. Lawrence, A. M.: Glucagon in medicine: new ideas for an old hormone. Med. Clin. North Am., *54*:183, 1970.
73. Lawrence, A. M.: Glucagon. Annu. Rev. Med., *20*:207, 1969.
74. Lefebvre, P. J., Luyckx, A. S., and Nizet, A. H.: Renal handling of endogenous glucagon in the dog: comparison with insulin. Metabolism, *23*:753, 1974.
75. Mann, R. J.: Historical vignette "honey urine" to pancreatic diabetes: 600 B.C.-1922. Mayo Clin. Proc., *46*:56, 1971.
76. Manns, J. G., and Martin, C. L.: Plasma insulin, glucagon, and nonesterified fatty acids in dogs with diabetes mellitus. Am. J. Vet. Res., *33*:981, 1972.
77. Mayhew, D. A., Wright, P. H., and Ashmore, J.: Regulation of insulin secretion. Pharmacol. Rev., *21*:183, 1969.
78. Mitchell, M. L., et al.: Detection of growth-hormone deficiency. New Engl. J. Med., *282*:539, 1970.
79. Ninomiya, R., et al.: Effect of adrenal steroids on glucose kinetics in normal and diabetic dogs. Diabetes, *14*:729, 1965.
80. Ohneda, A., et al.: Suppression of pancreatic glucagon secretion by tolbutamide in dogs. Horm. Metab. Res., *6*:477, 1974.
81. Orci, L.: A portrait of the pancreatic B-cell. Diabetologia *10*:163, 1974.
82. Ota, K., et al.: Endocrine function of the pancreatic allograft. Endocrinology, *82*:731, 1968.
83. Patz, A., et al.: Studies on diabetic retinopathy. Diabetes, *14*:700, 1965.
84. Pingel, M., Vølund, A., and Techn, L.: Stability of insulin preparations. Diabetes, *21*:805, 1972.
85. Porte, D., Jr., and Bagdade, J. D.: Human insulin secretion: an integrated approach. Annu. Rev. Med., *21*:219, 1970.
86. Prout, T. E.: A prospective view of the treatment of adult-onset diabetes. Med. Clin. North Am., *55*:1065, 1971.
87. Ravel, R.: Current methods for diagnosing diabetes mellitus. Postgrad. Med., *42*:40, 1967.
88. Rerup, C. C.: Drugs producing diabetes through damage of the insulin secreting cells. Pharmacol. Rev., *22*:485, 1970.
89. Rimoin, D. L.: Inheritance in diabetes mellitus. Med. Clin. North Am., *55*:807, 1971.
90. Root, C. R., and Scott, R. C.: Emphysematous cystitis and other radiographic manifestations of diabetes mellitus in dogs and cats. J. Am. Vet. Med. Assoc., *158*:721, 1971.
91. Ross, J. R., Warren, K. W., and Rudolph, N. E.: Zollinger-Ellison syndrome. Med. Clin. North Am., *50*:469, 1966.
92. Roth, H., Thier, S., and Segal, S.: Zinc glucagon in the management of refractory hypoglycemia due to insulin-producing tumors. New Engl. J. Med., *274*:493, 1966.

93. Rouse, B. T., and Wilson, M. R.: A case of hypoglycaemia in a dog associated with neoplasia of the pancreas. Vet. Rec., *79*:454, 1966.
94. Rubenstein, A. H., and Steiner, D. F.: Proinsulin. Med. Clin. North Am., *54*:191, 1970.
95. Rynearson, E. H.: True hyperinsulinism versus functional hypoglycemia. Postgrad. Med., *32*:189, 1962.
96. Singer, M. M.: Endocrine emergencies. Med. Clin. North Am., *55*:1315, 1971.
97. Smith, L. F.: Amino acid sequences of insulins. Diabetes, *21*:457, 1972.
98. Smith, L. F.: Species variation in the amino acid sequence of insulin. Am. J. Med., *40*:662, 1966.
99. Sokal, J. E., Lowe, C. U., and Sarcione, E. J.: Liver glycogen disease. Arch. Intern. Med., *109*:158, 1962.
100. Steinke, J.: Management of diabetes in the surgical patient. Med. Clin. North Am., *55*:939, 1971.
101. Steinke, J., and Taylor, K. W.: Viruses and the etiology of diabetes. Diabetes, *23*:631, 1974.
102. Strafuss, A. C., et al.: Islet call neoplasm in four dogs. J. Am. Vet. Med. Assoc., *159*:1008, 1971.
103. Thornton, G. F.: Infections and diabetes. Med. Clin. North Am., *55*:931, 1971.
104. Tischler, S. A.: The effect of the estrous cycle on diabetes mellitus in the dog. J. Am. Anim. Hosp. Assoc., *10*:122, 1974.
105. Tomhave, W. G.: Treatment of diabetes mellitus with oral hypoglycemic compounds. Med. Clin. North Am., *47*:53, 1963.
106. Tyson, J. E.: Obstetrical management of the pregnant diabetic. Med. Clin. North Am., *55*:961, 1971.
107. Tyson, J. E.: Medical aspects of diabetes in pregnancy and the diabetogenic effects of oral contraceptives. Med. Clin. North Am., *55*:947, 1971.
108. Unger, R. H., and Orci, L.: The essential role of glucagon in the pathogenesis of diabetes mellitus. Lancet, *1*:14, 1975.
109. Unger, R. H.: Insulin/glucagon ratio. Isr. J. Med. Sci., *8*:252, 1972.
110. Unger, R. H.: Glucagon and the insulin:glucagon ratio in diabetes and other catabolic illnesses. Diabetes, *20*:834, 1971.
111. Walker, D.: Diabetes mellitus following steroid therapy in a dog. Vet. Rec., *74*:1543, 1962.
112. Watts, C.: Failure of an impregnated cellulose strip as a test for glucose in urine. Vet. Rec., *32*:48, 1968.
113. Way, L., Goldman, L., and Dunphy, J. E.: Zollinger-Ellison syndrome. Am. J. Surg., *116*:293, 1968.
114. Wiertz-Hoessels, E. L. M. J.: Histologische und histochemische Veränderungen des Pancreas in zwei Fällen Diabetes mellitus bei Hunden. Zentralbl. Veterinaermed., *8*:687, 1966.
115. Williamson, J. R., Volger, N. J., and Kilo, C.: Microvascular disease in diabetes. Med. Clin. North Am., *55*:847, 1971.
116. Wilson, R. B., and Wilson, W. D.: Hepatotoxicity of tolbutamide in dogs. J. Am. Vet. Med. Assoc., *156*:1557, 1970.
117. Winegrad, A. I., and Clements, R. S., Jr.: Diabetic ketoacidosis. Med. Clin. North Am., *55*:899, 1971.
118. Zaharko, D. S., Beck, L. V., and Blankenbaker, R.: Role of the kidney in the disposal of radioiodinated and nonradioiodinated insulin in dogs. Diabetes, *15*:680, 1966.

Chapter

10

The Adrenal Cortex

The adrenal glands comprise two separate anatomic and functional units, the cortex and the medulla. These two parts have different developmental origins; in fact, in the fish, for example, the adrenal cortex and medulla occur as separate glands. In the dog the medulla, which is derived from ectodermal tissue, is incorporated within and surrounded by the cortex, which is derived from mesodermal tissue.

ANATOMY

The adrenal glands are two somewhat flattened and triangular structures located craniad and mediad to the anterior poles of the kidneys. The right gland lies between the medial surface of the anterior pole of the right kidney and the lateral aspect of the vena cava. The left gland lies mediad to the anterior pole of the left kidney. The blood supply reaches the adrenal glands through a number of short arterioles, which enter the gland mainly through the dorsal surface. Venous drainage is almost completely through a single vein.

Three different types of zones are formed by the cell structure of the cortex. Immediately beneath the capsule of the gland are the parenchymal cells, which are grouped into small irregular clusters with capillaries lying between them. This area, comprising about 25% of the cortex, is the *zona glomerulosa.* Since in the dog these clusters may take on a sigmoid or U-shaped arrangement, this area is also called the zona arcuata. Beneath this outer zone is the *zona fasciculata,* where the cells are arranged in somewhat regular and straight cords running at right angles to the surface of the capsule. This area comprises approximately 60% of the cortex. The innermost zone, comprising 15% of the cortex and lying adjacent to the medulla, is the *zona reticularis*. The cells in this area are arranged in somewhat anastomosing cords that appear to run in a number of different directions.

PHYSIOLOGY

Basic Chemistry of Steroids

The steroids are organic compounds containing the perhydrocyclopentanophenanthrene nucleus. Included in this group are cholesterol, the androgens, the estrogens, the adrenocortical hormones, progesterone, and the metabolites of these compounds.

The steroid nucleus contains 17 carbon atoms. The androgens have two angular methyl groups attached to the nucleus, one at C-10 and the other at C-13, giving them a 19-carbon-atom molecular structure. The estrogens, on the other hand, do not contain an angular methyl group at C-10, and therefore have only 18 carbon atoms. An unsaturated phenolic ring structure is present in the estrogens. Progesterone and the adrenocortical steroids are C-21 structures having a two-carbon chain attached at C-17.

Corticosteroids

The adrenal cortex secretes estrogens, androgens, probably some progesterone, and corticosteroids. The latter group affects intermediate metabolism of carbohydrate, protein, and fat, and also influences the distribution of water and electrolytes. The corticosteroids are further classified as glucocorticoids or mineralocorticoids, depending on their primary function.

Large numbers of corticosteroids have been isolated from adrenocortical tissue, most of these being intermediates that are not normally secreted to any extent into the circulation. Present evidence suggests that the principal adrenocortical hormones are cortisol, corticosterone, and aldosterone. Cortisol, the major glucocorticoid, is the steroid that is mainly involved in the negative feedback mechanism on the control of ACTH secretion. This steroid exerts its influence on corticotropin-releasing factor (CRF) in the hypothalamus. Aldosterone is the principal mineralocorticoid, and corticosterone has both glucocorticoid and mineralocorticoid activity.

The secretion of cortisol is not constant throughout the day. The circadian rhythm of cortisol and ACTH secretion fluctuates from one day to another. Maximal cortisol secretion occurs late in the day, with the peak level occurring between midnight and early morning. Both ACTH activity and cortisol secretion gradually decrease during the day, and by late evening cortisol secretion is at its minimum.

The biologic activity of the steroidal hormones depends on the effective concentration in the serum, that is, the amount of the particular steroid that is free and available at the tissue level. Cortisol, similar to other steroids, is carried in the blood partially bound to certain plasma proteins. Most of the unconjugated cortisol in plasma is bound to an alpha globulin, transcortin; to a lesser extent, some cortisol is bound to albumin. In man transcortin increases appreciably in the latter stages of pregnancy or under the influence of estrogen therapy. In addition, transcortin levels decrease in conditions that are characterized by abnormalities of serum proteins.

The glucocorticoids, in addition to their activity on glucose homeostasis, are the compounds possessing anti-inflammatory activity. The glucocorticoids possess other biologic activities affecting cytologic processes and intermediate metabolism. They are catabolic, and thus tend to produce a negative nitrogen balance. They also produce a negative calcium balance by increasing the excretion of calcium in the urine and inhibiting the absorption of calcium in the intestinal tract. This latter action appears to be mediated through an inhibitory action on vitamin D.

Steroidogenesis

The corticosteroids are derived from cholesterol, which originally arises from acetate. Cleavage of a segment of the cholesterol side chain produces an intermediate compound, pregnenolone. This reaction appears to be under the influence of ACTH, since in its absence, only about 10% of the normal biosynthesis of the steroid hormones takes place. Based on the intermediate steroids that have

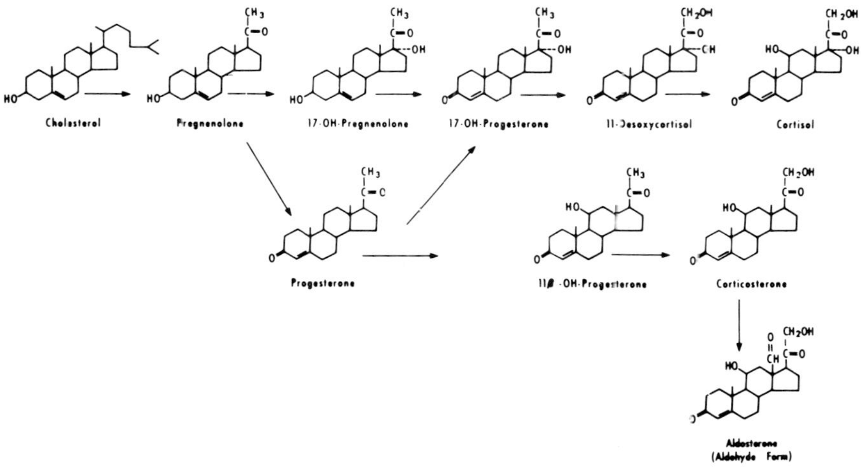

Fig. 10–1. Proposed corticosteroid biosynthesis in the canine adrenal gland. (From Siegel, E. T.: Am. J. Vet. Res., *26*:1152, 1965.)

been isolated in the dog, both from adrenocortical tissue and in adrenal venous blood, a pathway for canine adrenocorticoid biosynthesis can be specified (Fig. 10–1).

Conversion of progesterone to cortisol involves important biologic hydroxylation, at C-17, 21, and 11, by the adrenocortical tissue, whereas the formation of corticosterone from progesterone involves hydroxylation at only C-11 and C-21. Corticosterone differs chemically from cortisol only by the absence of one hydroxy group at C-17. Although aldosterone biosynthesis is controlled by a different mechanism, it is essentially derived from corticosterone.

Catabolism of Steroids

The main biologic function of metabolism of the steroid hormones is to remove the active hormones from the animal. In general, the major site for metabolic degradation of all steroid hormones is the liver. Although part of the metabolic activity takes place in peripheral tissues, it is minor in comparison to the liver.

In the dog, following administration of radioactively labeled cortisol, the following catabolites have been isolated in the urine: labeled cortol, 3-epiallocortol, cortolone, 3-epiallotetrahydrocortisol, and tetrahydrocortisol. These catabolites are excreted mainly as glucuronides, and a major portion of this fraction is represented by steroids that are reduced at C-20 (Fig. 10–2). Since these catabolites are reduced at C-20, the use of steroid assay procedures that measure only those steroids having a dihydroxyketolic side-chain, such as the Porter-Silber reaction, would not measure these cortisol catabolites in the dog. In assessing urinary steroids in the dog, it is helpful to use

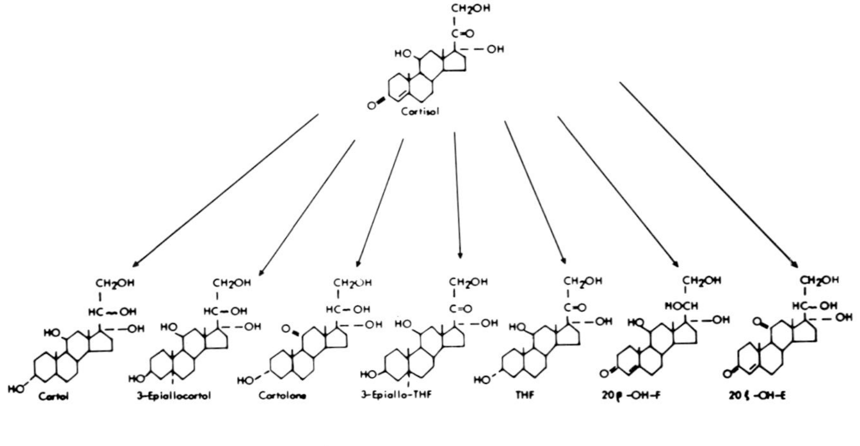

Fig. 10–2. In vivo cortisol metabolism in the dog. (From Siegel, E. T.: Am. J. Vet. Res., *20*:1152, 1965.)

methods that quantitate compounds with the dihydroxyketolic side-chain plus those catabolites with the further reduced side-chain. This assessment is easily accomplished using a 17-ketogenic steroid (17-KGS) assay procedure, which shows that the urinary excretion of these steroids in normal mature dogs is 2.08 ± 0.70 mg/24 hours, with a range between 1.13 and 3.67 mg/24 hours. Intramuscular administration of ACTH gel causes an increase of these steroids in urinary excretions, ranging between 0.14 and 3.97 mg/24 hours, with a mean increase of 1.64 mg/24 hours.

Regulation of Glucocorticoid Secretion

In the complete absence of ACTH, there is still a small (perhaps 10%) basal secretion of glucocorticoids. Most glucocorticoid secretion is controlled by ACTH secretion from the anterior pituitary. Normally, a basal secretion of ACTH is maintained, showing a diurnal variation. The origin of the original stimulus to this diurnal secretion of ACTH is undoubtedly the release of corticotropin-releasing factor (CRF). The further controlling mechanism of CRF is located within the central nervous system. This basal diurnal level of ACTH stimulates sufficient corticosteroids to supply the permissive needs of the animal, and also keeps the adrenal gland sufficiently large and responsive in case further stressful situations require corticosteroid output.

Normally, as cortisol levels increase in the blood in response to the need of the animal, they inhibit the release of CRF in the hypothalamus when a certain level is exceeded. As a result, there is less secretion of ACTH. This feedback mechanism is important in maintaining physiologic levels of circulating cortisol.

During periods of acute stress in which corticosteroid secretion is necessary, the release of CRF-ACTH will not adequately increase this secretion if its prior release has not effected normal levels. Adrenal size and responsiveness under these conditions would be decreased. This problem in the cycle explains why animals on long-term corticosteroid therapy respond poorly to stress. The corticosteroid therapy produces a somewhat prolonged and continued adrenocortical atrophy. Like cortisol, exogenous corticosteroids, when administered to an animal, depress ACTH release. The animal on long-term therapy has an atrophied adrenal gland but no signs of adrenocortical insufficiency, since the exogenous corticosteroids take the place of the normal endogenous secretions. In addition, aldosterone secretion is not affected, since aldosterone is not primarily controlled through ACTH stimulation.

Difficulties associated with glucocorticoid administration occur when the adrenal gland remains atrophic after discontinuance of the exogenous steroids. In the dog this gland atrophy is only a minor problem, which is dependent on the amount of exogenous steroid administered and the length of time of administration. The continued adrenocortical atrophy, after discontinuation of exogenous steroid administration, appears to be related to nonresumption of the normal diurnal release of CRF. This adrenocortical atrophy can be avoided by decreasing the exogenous steroid gradually, so that the secretion of CRF and ACTH can resume.

In primary adrenal insufficiency, when cortisol secretion is decreased, there is a marked increase in ACTH secretion. The basic feedback mechanism involves a reciprocal relationship between cortisol and ACTH secretion. When cortisol secretion is higher than normal, ACTH level is depressed; if the cortisol level is depressed, ACTH secretion is increased. The only exception to this reciprocal relationship occurs during periods of stress, in which both ACTH and cortisol are maintained at a higher level. Under stress, higher centers within the CNS are able to override the negative feedback mechanism. There appear to be different levels of suppressibility of ACTH secretion based on the secretion of different CRF controlling factors. Under nonstressful conditions CRF mainly stimulates the control of the diurnal mechanism. This particular CRF is easily suppressed using exogenous corticosteroids. However, the CRF secreted during stress is relatively nonsuppressible with normal quantities of corticosteroids. The dual CRF control may explain the differences in suppressibility of ACTH secretion seen with different adrenocortical disorders.

Biologic Actions of Glucocorticoids

The glucocorticoids affect carbohydrate, protein, and calcium metabolism, inflammation, blood pressure, and certain hematologic elements. Glucocorticoids affect carbohydrate metabolism in a number of different ways. These steroids inhibit the peripheral utilization of glucose — the so-called "anti-insulin effect." In addition, the glucocorticoids increase the production of liver glycogen, and they stimulate gluconeogenesis. Although administration of glucocorticoids in the dog does increase gluconeogenesis, it does not increase the blood glucose concentration. This result is in contrast to the hyperglycemia that can be produced in other species through administration of these steroids. The suggestion is that, as the increased gluconeogenesis occurs, the canine pancreas is able to increase the secretion of insulin in a compensatory manner to prevent the development of hyperglycemia. However, even though acute administration of steroids in the dog does not produce hyperglycemia, long-term administration of glucocorticoids in this species can produce steroid diabetes. Since dogs with Cushing's syndrome accompanied by increased endogenous glucocorticoid levels also have increased insulin secretion, it seems likely that steroid diabetes results when the pancreas is no longer able to secrete the necessary amount of insulin; the pancreas then goes into "exhaustion atrophy."

The hematologic changes associated with glucocorticoids are mainly a decrease in circulating lymphocytes and eosinophils, and a slight increase in neutrophils. The effect on the neutrophils is relatively less pronounced than the effect on the eosinophils and lymphocytes. A number of years ago, one assay procedure for adrenal function was based on the ability of the glucocorticoids to produce an eosinopenia. Although the eosinopenia produced is a fairly sensitive indication of glucocorticoid action, this type of assay procedure is not considered to be a reliable index of adrenal function.

Small amounts of glucocorticoids are necessary as permissive hormones for protein metabolism. When glucocorticoids become excessive, they produce a catabolic effect on protein metabolism. In canine hyperadrenocorticalism the protein catabolic effect of the steroids produces a characteristic change in the skin due to the breakdown of collagen and elastic fibers. Glucocorticoids, therefore, produce a negative nitrogen balance if they are secreted in excessive amounts.

Glucocorticoids also affect calcium metabolism. These steroids can produce a negative calcium balance by inhibiting the absorption of calcium in the gut, and by increasing the excretion of calcium in the urine. The inhibiting effect on gastrointestinal absorption of calcium appears to be mediated through an inhibition of the action of vitamin D. In hyperadrenocorticalism or with long-term administration of excessive glucocorticoids, this negative calcium balance eventually leads to the development of osteoporosis. However, with excessive glucocorticoids the serum calcium level is normal if parathyroid function is unaltered. The negative calcium balance stimulates a compensatory increased secretion of parathormone, which leads to removal of calcium from bone and the maintenance of normocalcemia.

Blood pressure control is partially under the influence of the glucocorticoids. The glucocorticoids contribute to a normal blood pressure through a synergistic effect with norepinephrine. In adrenalectomized dogs maintained on adequate amounts of mineralocorticoids only, the blood pressure is lower than normal. Following glucocorticoid administration, the blood pressure returns to normal levels rapidly.

Glucocorticoids inhibit inflammation and delay wound healing. Because of the former effect, they are a common therapy for inflammatory disease. With hyperadrenocorticalism and excessive endogenous glucocorticoids, inflammation is also suppressed and wound healing delayed.

Control of Aldosterone Secretion

The mechanism regulating the production and release of aldosterone is different from the one for control and secretion of cortisol. Located around the afferent arterioles leading to the glomeruli in the kidney is a group of cells called the juxtaglomerular cells (Fig. 10–3). Present experimental evidence has focused on the importance of the circulating plasma volume perfusing the arterial system of the renal glomeruli. During dehydration, when plasma volume decreases, renin substrate (angiotensinogen), a circulating precursor of angiotensin, is converted to angiotensin-I by renin. The latter is synthesized and stored in the juxtaglomerular cells. Angiotensinogen is produced

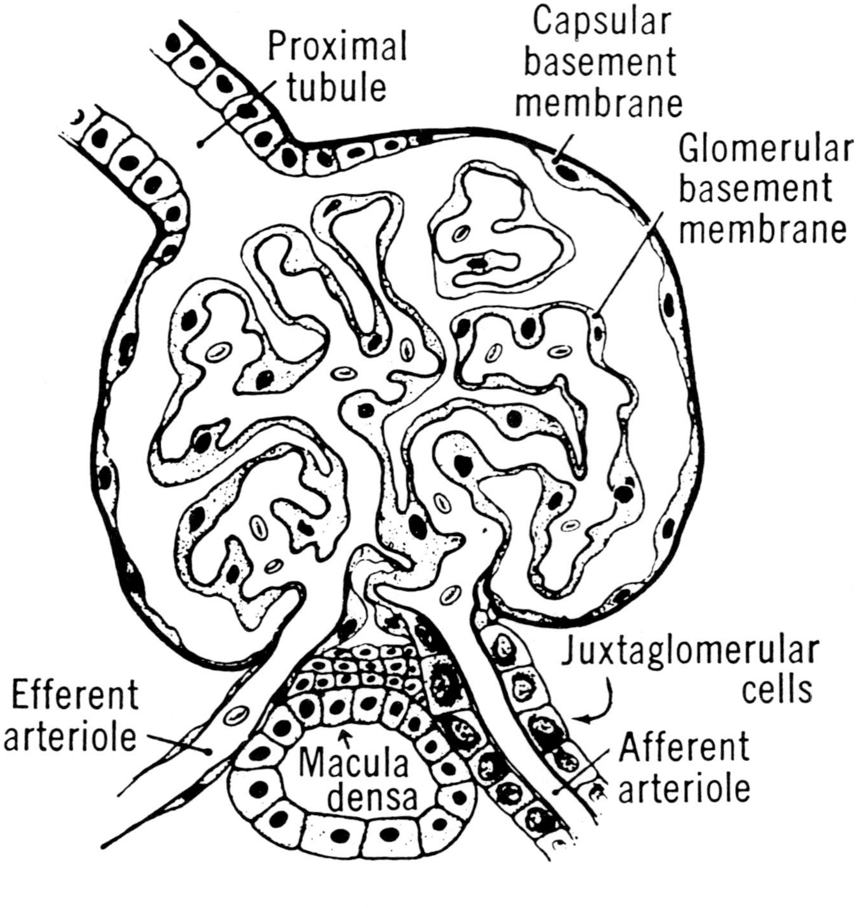

Fig. 10–3. Relationship of the juxtaglomerular cells and the macula densa to the glomerulus and its circulation. (From Gordon, E. S.: Postgrad. Med., *40*:138, 1966.)

in the liver, and is a polypeptide associated with, or incorporated into, an α-2 globulin circulating in the blood. Angiotensin-I, a decapeptide, is rapidly converted into angiotensin-II, an octapeptide, by the action of a converting enzyme in plasma. Angiotensin-II stimulates the production and release of aldosterone from the zona glomerulosa.

An additional group of cells, the macula densa, may be involved with the physiologic control of aldosterone secretion. This cell group, an element of the distal tubule, makes contact with the vascular pole of its own glomerulus, and is attached to the juxtaglomerular cells of the afferent glomerular arteriole. The macula densa may act as a sensing element to relate changes in release of renin to a distal renal tubular event, such as a change in sodium concentration or sodium load, bulk flow of tubular fluid, or osmolality of tubular fluid.

Biologic Actions of Aldosterone

Aldosterone enhances the excretion of potassium and increases reabsorption of sodium by the kidney. Although evidence is conflicting, the major site of action of aldosterone appears to be the distal tubule of the kidney. This effect on sodium and potassium metabolism is not dependent on either a change in the glomerular filtration rate or other extratubular effects. The increased reabsorption of sodium is accompanied by an increased reabsorption of water. In addition to enhancing the excretion of potassium into the urine, aldosterone influences the excretion of hydrogen ions. The excretion of sodium and potassium does not appear to be affected by a simple exchange mechanism.

Aldosterone has a supporting role in maintaining blood pressure through its action on sodium retention and thus on plasma volume control. However, it is far less important in maintaining blood pressure than the glucocorticoids. During adrenal crisis, aldosterone fails to restore blood pressure, vigor, or even electrolyte concentrations in the plasma of adrenalectomized dogs, whereas glucocorticoids have a very supportive role on the blood pressure in adrenal crisis.

The role of aldosterone in sodium and potassium metabolism is less important in tissues other than the kidney, i.e., the sweat glands, the salivary glands, and the intestines.

LABORATORY TESTS

Recent years have brought much improvement in the laboratory tests used for evaluating adrenocortical diseases. At one time assay techniques were long and laborious procedures requiring relatively large amounts of hormone for quantitation. With the development of radioimmunoassay procedures, the sensitivity of the techniques has increased, and now minute amounts of hormones can be assayed.

Urinary Steroids

Measurement of adrenocortical steroids and their metabolites in the urine can be carried out utilizing chemical assay techniques. Although 24-hour collection of urine is necessary, often milligram quantities of steroids can be isolated. In addition, other recent procedures can measure groups of steroids, i.e., compounds with similar chemical structures.

Urinary 17-hydroxycorticosteroids may be determined by a number of different methods. These procedures measure C-21 compounds, excluding the progestational compounds, and therefore are somewhat useful for assessment of adrenocortical steroids. A common procedure uses the Porter-Silber reaction, which quantitates steroids having a 17, 21-dihydroxy-20-ketone side-chain. Since cortisol and some of its catabolites have this type of chemical structure, this technique is useful for evaluating adrenocortical function. However, limitations do exist. Since the dog catabolizes cortisol mainly to compounds that have a further reduced side-chain (17,20,21-trihydroxysteroids), these compounds would not be quantitated using the Porter-Silber reaction. Therefore, the usual 17-hydroxycorticosteroid determination method using the Porter-Silber reaction does not quantitate a significant percentage of the catabolites of cortisol.

Although 17-hydroxycorticosteroid determination using the Porter-Silber reaction is less than satisfactory for canine urine, another type of procedure is useful. Using a 17-ketogenic steroid assay procedure, the cortisol catabolites with a dihydroxy-ketone side-chain are assayed as are those catabolites with the further reduced side-chain. The 17-ketogenic steroid assay quantitates most of the catabolites of cortisol in canine urine.

Another procedure once used for assessing adrenal function in man is the 17-ketosteroid assay. This procedure measures C-19 compounds having a keto-group at the C-17 position. Some corticosteroids in man are catabolized to 17-ketosteroids, and some of these ketosteroids are weak androgens or catabolites of androgens. ACTH administration increases the secretion of 17-ketosteroids in man. In the dog this assay has not been useful for assessing adrenocortical function. Although 17-ketosteroids are present in canine urine, the origin of these compounds is unknown, and they do not respond to ACTH stimulation.

Additional chemical techniques are available for measuring either specific steroids or groups of steroids. While these techniques were useful before the era of the radioimmunoassay, they required collection of complete 24-hour samples. With today's more sensitive techniques, it is possible to measure hormones directly in biologic fluids or tissues.

Plasma Steroids

Since cortisol is the major glucocorticoid and aldosterone the major mineralocorticoid, the development of techniques to measure these steroids has increased the knowledge of adrenocortical disorders.

At present a sensitive technique for radioimmunoassay of plasma cortisol is particularly useful for evaluating adrenocortical function if used with a stimulatory or suppression test.

Secretion of some of the plasma steroids exhibits a diurnal variation. Plasma cortisol levels reach their minimum in the circulation near midnight. At approximately 2 A.M., the plasma cortisol level begins to increase, reaching its maximum near 8 A.M. During the rest of the day, there is a progressive decrease in the plasma cortisol level. The normal plasma cortisol level in the dog ranges from less than 1.0 to 4.0 μg%. Since a normal plasma level of less than 1.0 μg% is possible, the low values seen with adrenocortical insufficiency cannot be differentiated using this technique. To overcome this difficulty, a stimulation test can be used.

The determination of aldosterone in plasma is also possible. However, this technique is not as readily available as is the plasma cortisol determination. The cost of aldosterone determinations presently inhibits the usefulness of this procedure in veterinary practice.

Secretion Rates

An accurate assessment of adrenal function can be made using a specific secretion rate determination. This technique involves the infusion of a radioactive steroid, as well as the isolation and quantitation of the radioactive steroid and its catabolites in the urine. Using this type of procedure, one can determine the amount of the particular steroid that is secreted over a 24-hour period. However, the difficulty of infusing a radioactive substance over a number of hours, the collection of the urine over a period of time, and the handling of the samples make this type of procedure impractical for clinical practice.

ACTH Stimulation Tests

The availability of a synthetic ACTH preparation (Cortrosyn) has improved the technique for assessing adrenocortical function. Using a 1-24 adrenocorticotropic hormone (ACTH) in conjunction with the radioimmunoassay for cortisol, adrenocortical function can be accurately evaluated.

In the normal dog weighing 10 pounds or more, 0.125 mg of synthetic ACTH injected intramuscularly increases the plasma cortisol up to 6.0 μg% over the preinjection level in 30 minutes. In dogs under 10 pounds of body weight, 0.0625 mg of the synthetic ACTH should be injected. In the dog with primary adrenocortical insufficiency the preinjection cortisol level is low and results in little or no response to ACTH. With hyperfunctional disease of the adrenal cortex, the ACTH stimulation test is useful for differentiating bilateral adrenocortical hyperplasia from neoplasia. Usually with hyperplastic adrenocortical disease the administration of synthetic ACTH produces an exaggerated plasma cortisol response, in many cases three- to five-fold greater than the preinjection level. With adrenocortical neoplasia, the plasma cortisol level usually is higher than the normal preinjection level, but the response to synthetic ACTH is minimal or absent.

Dexamethasone Suppression Test

A suppression test depends on the substitution of a synthetic analog or drug to inhibit the secretion of a specific hormone. For evaluating certain adrenocortical diseases, the potent glucocorticoid, dexamethasone, has been used because it can successfully suppress cortisol secretion. In man use of this test is based on the fact that a specific oral dose (0.5 mg) of dexamethasone administered every six hours results in a decrease in plasma cortisol within one or two days in normal people. However, this same dose of dexamethasone does not significantly decrease the plasma cortisol in patients with Cushing's syndrome. The technique has been further refined so that different doses of dexamethasone will cause suppression. Higher levels of dexamethasone (2.0 mg every six hours) do suppress cortisol secretion in patients with bilateral adrenocortical hyperplasia. However, even the higher dose of dexamethasone does not suppress cortisol secretion in patients with neoplasms of either the adrenal cortex or the anterior pituitary.

Although a dexamethasone suppression test would probably be of value in the dog, the optimal doses have not been worked out. Despite reports of dexamethasone suppression tests in the dog, this technique needs further refinement before definite conclusions can be based on the results.

Metyrapone Test for ACTH Reserve

Metyrapone (2-methyl-1,2-di-3-pyridyl-1-propanone) is a drug that successfully inhibits the 11-β hydroxylation of steroids by adrenocortical tissue. Since this compound inhibits enzymatic hydroxylation, it results in the formation of 11-desoxycortisol while preventing the formation of cortisol. The resulting decreased level of cortisol leads to less feedback control on the hypothalamus, and thus an increased secretion of CRF. This change produces a corresponding increase in ACTH. In using this test, response to the drug can be assessed

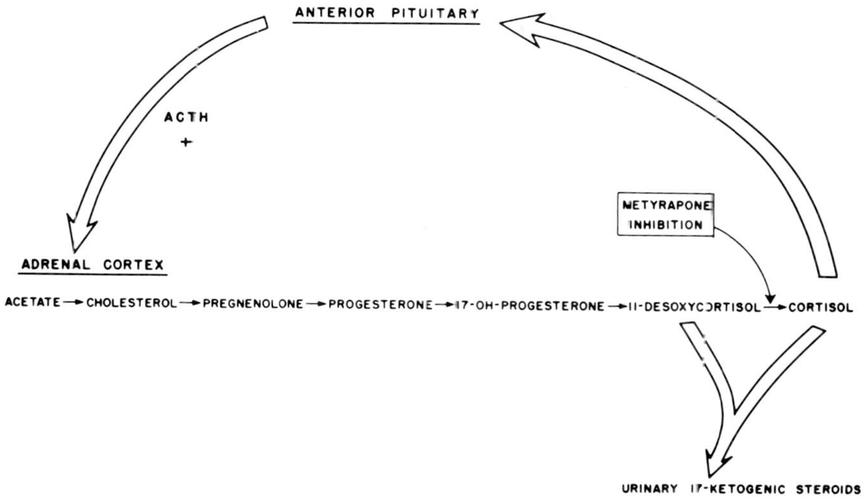

Fig. 10–4. Evaluation of residual adrenocorticotropin (ACTH) reserve in the pituitary gland. The response to metyrapone may be assessed by evaluation of serum levels of ACTH or 11-desoxycortisol, and/or urinary levels of 17-ketogenic steroids. (From Siegel, E. T.: Am. J. Vet. Res., *29*:173, 1968.)

directly by radioimmunoassay of ACTH, or indirectly by measurement of 11-desoxycortisol or its catabolites in the urine. Since in the dog, 11-desoxycortisol is catabolized to compounds that are assessed using the 17-ketogenic steroid assay procedure, this technique can be used to follow the response to metyrapone administration (Fig. 10–4). This technique has been reported for assessing pituitary adrenocortical function in the dog, but its usefulness is rather limited.

HYPOFUNCTION — ADRENAL INSUFFICIENCY

A clinical syndrome associated with the destruction of the adrenal glands was first described in 1849 by Thomas Addison. The resulting adrenal insufficiency, which he also described, is still commonly called Addison's disease. Specifically, Addison's disease is more closely termed a chronic adrenal insufficiency due to extensive destruction of the adrenal cortex. Another cause of adrenocortical insufficiency, but not necessarily considered Addison's disease, is the atrophy of the adrenal cortex induced by administration of exogenous steroids. Acute adrenal insufficiency can also occur in association with massive hemorrhage into the adrenal cortices, often associated with certain types of septicemias. This latter type of acute adrenal insufficiency has been termed Waterhouse-Friderichsen syndrome in man.

Etiology

Primary adrenal insufficiency can result from any destructive lesion affecting the adrenal cortices bilaterally. This insufficiency may result from autoimmune adrenocortical atrophy, massive hemorrhage into the adrenals, bilateral adrenocortical metastases, amyloidosis, or any other infiltrative and destructive disease affecting both adrenal glands.

Extensive adrenocortical atrophy is present in appproximately 90% of the cases of primary adrenal insufficiency in the dog. Although the cause of this specific lesion was unknown for many years, its histologic appearance is consistent with that of an autoimmune disease. Some recent experimental evidence strongly supports the hypothesis that adrenocortical atrophy is caused by an autoimmune disorder. The affected adrenals have a histologic appearance similar to other tissues with autoimmune disease, i.e., infiltration of lymphocytes and round cells, fibrosis, and atrophy of the epithelial cells. In addition, specific antibodies against adrenocortical cells have been found in the circulation. Antibodies against other tissues, particularly the thyroid, have also been found associated with immunoadrenocortical atrophy in man. Finally, similar lesions can be produced in experimental animals by injection of autologous adrenal tissue in Freund's adjuvant.

Acute adrenal insufficiency may result when hemorrhage into the adrenal cortices is extensive. This type of disorder occurs in association with certain septicemias in children. In the dog a similar type of adrenal insufficiency is seen on occasion. Occasionally lymphosarcoma or other neoplastic disease may involve the adrenals bilaterally, sufficiently replacing the normal tissue and producing signs of adrenocortical insufficiency. Metastatic tumors on rare occasions can produce a similar situation. Amyloidosis, although rare, may produce adrenocortical insufficiency by depositing amyloid within the adrenal cortex. The amyloid causes massive destruction of the adrenocortical tissue.

Primary adrenocortical insufficiency due to the autoimmune disorder is commonly seen in dogs under five years of age, with most affected animals being between one and three years of age. In contrast, adrenocortical insufficiency in older dogs is more commonly associated with lesions, such as bilateral adrenocortical neoplasia or amyloidosis. Although these lesions are the ones usually seen, any abnormality that results in infiltration or destruction of the adrenal cortices, if extensive enough, may produce primary adrenal insufficiency.

Pathologic Findings

The most characteristic finding in dogs with primary adrenal insufficiency is massive destruction of the adrenal cortices. In

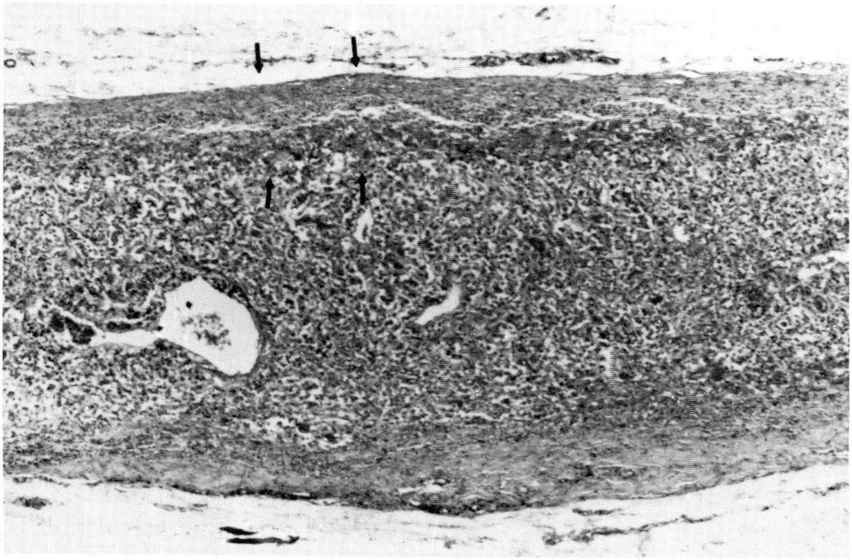

Fig. 10–5. Adrenocortical atrophy ×34. The cortex is greatly reduced in size, and there is almost complete lack of normal architecture present. (Courtesy John T. McGrath, University of Pennsylvania.)

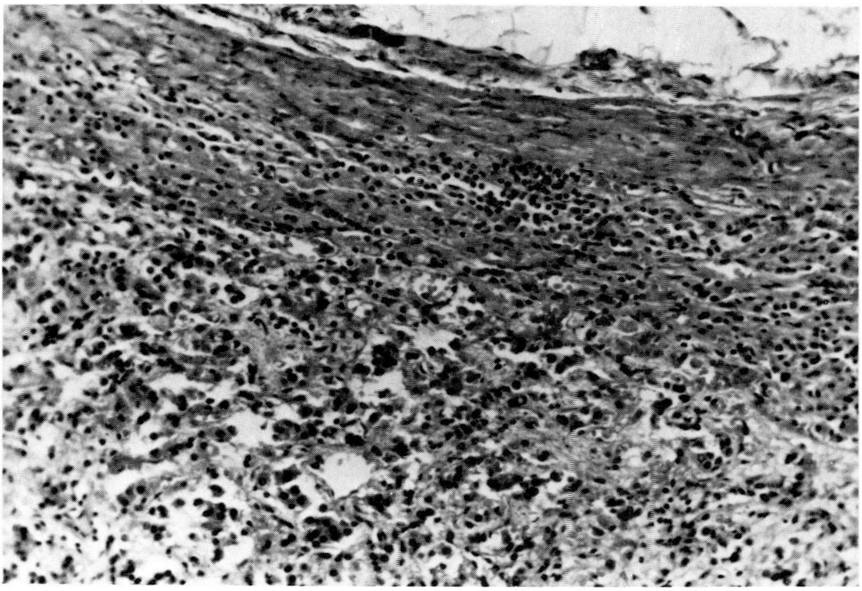

Fig. 10–6. Adrenocortical atrophy ×102. There is marked cellular infiltration into the atrophied cortex. The cells are predominately lymphocytes with occasional plasma cells. (Courtesy John T. McGrath, University of Pennsylvania.)

adrenocortical atrophy, the normal architecture of the cortex is disrupted (Fig. 10–5), and there is massive infiltration of the tissue with lymphocytes and plasma cells (Fig. 10–6). If the adrenocortical atrophy is well developed, the zona glomerulosa, fasciculata, and reticularis are not discernible.

Chronic Phase

Theoretically, adrenocortical insufficiency may be caused by primary disease within the adrenal cortex, or it may be secondary to hypothalamic-pituitary failure. In pituitary or secondary adrenocortical insufficiency, the defect is primarily a deficiency of ACTH, so it results mainly in a decreased secretion of cortisol. The dog is able to function fairly well with only mineralocorticoids present, but, with an ACTH insufficiency where the renin-angiotensin-aldosterone system is intact, the animal does not have pronounced clinical signs. Dogs appear to be able to maintain a relatively normal blood glucose and blood pressure in the absence of glucocorticoids (except probably during pronounced periods of stress). Therefore, secondary adrenocortical insufficiency is a minor clinical problem that is rarely diagnosed. It is seen in the dwarf with panhypopituitarism along with the other pituitary insufficiencies.

In primary adrenocortical insufficiency, the major clinical signs are those associated with an insufficiency of aldosterone. The clinical signs are related to the severity of the insufficiency of aldosterone, and usually the disorder is progressive. As the adrenal cortices begin to be destroyed, the secretion of aldosterone is compromised. With adrenocortical atrophy the adrenals appear to be destroyed over a protracted period of time, ranging from a few weeks to a few months. In young dogs with autoimmune adrenocortical insufficiency, the clinical signs of dehydration, emesis, diarrhea (which may be bloody), anorexia, and weakness may be present for one to four months. The increased pigmentation seen in man with adrenocortical insufficiency does not occur in the dog. The presence of hypotension and severe dehydration contributes to the development of the final crisis that occurs if the animal is untreated.

The most characteristic laboratory changes of primary adrenal insufficiency are those related to the electrolyte disturbance, that is, hyponatremia and hyperkalemia. The degree of change of these electrolytes is dependent on the severity and progression of the disease. The serum sodium level is usually below 135 mEq/L, and may even be lower than 120 mEq/L. The serum potassium level is usually greater than 5.5 mEq/L, but may be as high as 8 to 9 mEq/L. There is also an increase in circulating lymphocytes and eosinophils. However, this latter increase is not as constant a finding as the change in the serum sodium and potassium values. Occasionally the circulating eosinophils are as high as 15 to 20% of a differential CBC.

Adrenocortical insufficiency can be confirmed based on the plasma cortisol value before and after ACTH stimulation In the usual case, the preinjection plasma cortisol level is below 1 μg%, with little or no response to ACTH. Although this type of confirmatory test may be used, it is not usually necessary because of the diagnostic significance of the change in the electrolytes. When hyponatremia and hyperkalemia are present in an animal, it is reasonable to institute therapy for adrenal insufficiency rather than await final confirmation from the laboratory.

Another change possible with adrenocortical insufficiency is slight to moderate anemia. The anemia may be masked by the decrease in plasma volume and the resulting hemoconcentration. However, the total circulating red cell volume is decreased in some dogs with adrenal insufficiency. Other changes are acidosis and mild hypercalcemia.

Adrenocortical Crisis

Acute massive destruction of the adrenal cortices, or the terminal stage of progressive adrenocortical destruction, ends in adrenal crisis. In addition to the expected hyponatremia and hyperkalemia, this phase of adrenal insufficiency is characterized by severe hypotension, shock, hypoglycemia, and occasionally bradycardia. Adrenal crisis is a rapidly progressing and life-threatening situation. If untreated, it leads to death usually within 24 to 48 hours.

During an adrenal crisis the electrolyte changes are more pronounced than during the slowly developing chronic phase of adrenal insufficiency. Although the dog appears to be able to maintain its blood glucose level during the chronic phase of adrenal insufficiency, during the terminal adrenal crisis, hypoglycemia often develops. The dehydration and hypotension are due to the loss of intravascular fluids and sodium into the intracellular space as well as an extensive loss of water and sodium in the urine. Vascular dehydration may be greater than the loss in body weight. As a result of the severe dehydration and hypotension, prerenal azotemia develops.

Treatment

The specific therapy for adrenocortical insufficiency depends on whether one is treating an animal during an adrenal crisis or earlier, in the progressive and chronic phase of adrenal insufficiency. Treatment of adrenal crisis necessitates a vigorous type of therapy. The dog in adrenal crisis is also in renal failure. However, the activity of the mineralocorticoids depends on a functioning kidney, so it is absolutely necessary to establish urine flow as rapidly as possible. Initially saline solution with 5% dextrose is administered intravenously. Also a soluble corticosteroid is added to the intravenous fluids in an attempt to increase blood pressure and urine flow. For a medium-sized dog, 100 mg of cortisol hemisuccinate is administered in the first 250 ml of intravenous fluids. In addition to the intravenous therapy, a mineralocorticoid, desoxycorticosterone acetate (DOCA), is injected intramuscularly at a dose of 1 to 2 mg. The intramuscular administration of a glucocorticoid, such as 50 mg of cortisone acetate, is often given to supplement the intravenous administration.

During therapy of the adrenal crisis, the fluids and intravenous glucocorticoids are administered to effect. As the blood pressure increases, urine production is instituted, and within one to four hours after the beginning of the intravenous therapy, urine output is usually adequate. At this point, the mineralocorticoid administered becomes effective, resulting in the excretion of potassium into the urine and a decrease in the hyperkalemia. If continuous and severe shock with poor renal profusion persists, it may become necessary to administer additional vasopressor drugs. In most cases the administration of intravenous glucocorticoids in a saline and dextrose solution is sufficient to reverse the profound cardiovascular insufficiency. After renal function is restored, the clinical course becomes less life threatening, and the therapy is similar to that given in an early stage of progressing adrenal insufficiency.

Following recovery from an adrenal crisis, or beginning therapy with adrenal insufficiency but no crisis, the animal is given a daily administration of DOCA intramuscularly. Salt (0.5 to 1.0 g) is given orally in the food, and a glucocorticoid is administered either orally or intramuscularly until the animal is restored to a more normal state. After two days of therapy the serum sodium and potassium levels are rechecked to determine whether the dose of DOCA must be adjusted. The serum potassium level will be higher than normal and the serum sodium level lower than normal if the dose of DOCA is insufficient. If, however, excessive DOCA is administered, hypokalemia will develop. The dose of DOCA is adjusted until a normonatremia and normokalemia result.

After the animal is out of danger and its condition is somewhat stabilized, it is necessary to determine whether the adrenocortical insufficiency is permanent and requires lifelong treatment. With a temporary adrenocortical insufficiency, such as that occurring with adrenocortical hemorrhage, after therapy, the adrenal cortices may have enough functional tissue remaining so that regeneration occurs and lifelong treatment is not necessary. To establish whether the adrenocortical insufficiency is permanent, the clinician continues therapy for three to four weeks so that adrenocortical regeneration has time to occur. A long-acting mineralocorticoid, desoxycorticosterone

(DOC) pivalate, gives mineralocorticoid control for three to four weeks. A 25-mg intramuscular dose of the DOC pivalate releases the equivalent of 1 mg of DOCA per day. This length of time is necessary to establish whether the adrenal insufficiency is permanent. Following DOC pivalate administration, the animal is sent home, and usually only salt is added to the food daily. Occasionally an oral glucocorticoid, such as cortisol (5 mg/day), is also needed.

If the adrenal insufficiency is permanent, as the DOC pivalate effect decreases, the characteristic clinical and laboratory findings of adrenal insufficiency reappear. Three to four weeks after DOC pivalate treatment, hyponatremia and hyperkalemia redevelop, indicating that the adrenal insufficiency is permanent and therapy is needed for the lifetime of the animal. In those cases of nonpermanent adrenal insufficiency, the serum sodium and potassium levels remain normal after the four-week period. In the nonpermanent adrenal insufficient case, I recommend that electrolyte values be followed for an additional few weeks to be sure that adrenocortical function remains at normal levels.

For those animals needing lifetime maintenance therapy, fludrocortisone acetate tablets can be administered daily per os, or a local anesthetic can be used to implant a DOCA pellet under the skin in an area that will not be traumatized. This pellet releases DOCA for at least eight months since one 125-mg DOCA pellet releases 0.5 mg of DOCA per day. Although these pellets usually function for eight to twelve months, a monthly serum sodium and potassium level determination is necessary to evaluate the control with these pellets. As the pellet is becoming insufficient, the serum potassium level increases. As the serum potassium level increases above 5.2 mEq/L, additional pellets should be implanted.

After it is determined that the pellets have a specific functional life span, it is not necessary to check monthly electrolyte values after the second pellet implantation. Subsequent pellet implantation may be carried out at the determined time of their functional activity. The one exception to this rule is that, even if the serum sodium and potassium levels indicate that the pellets are functional after 11 months, additional pellets should be implanted at this time. I have found that the pellets in many of these dogs become insufficient between the eleventh and twelfth month. Rather than allow clinical signs to redevelop, with all the possible consequences, I recommend that pellets be implanted at this time.

For long-term therapy the owner usually has to administer only salt in the food each day. However, he should have on hand an oral glucocorticoid that can be administered if the animal is subjected to any undue stress. At this time 10 to 20 mg of cortisol per os can be administered twice daily. Occasionally an adrenal-insufficient dog appears to need small amounts of cortisol, 2.5 to 5.0 mg per os daily.

HYPERFUNCTIONAL ADRENOCORTICAL DISEASE

Pathological manifestations of oversecretion of any of the hormones produced by the adrenal cortex may occur. Although disease may involve secretion of more than one type of adrenocortical steroid, often the excessive secretion of one corticosteroid is mainly responsible for the characteristic and specific clinical syndrome. Hypercortisolism or Cushing's syndrome is the result of greater than normal secretion of cortisol; hyperaldosteronism is caused entirely by excessive secretion of aldosterone; and adrenal virilism results from the excessive production of androgens, either secreted by functional adrenal tumors or as the result of specific enzymatic defects of the adrenal cortex. Excessive androgen production secondary to an enzyme defect is called the adrenogenital syndrome. Last, although rare, is feminization due to estrogen-secreting neoplasia.

Cushing's Syndrome

Hypercortisolism or hypersecretion of glucocorticoids is the most common hyperfunctional disorder of the canine adrenal cortex. Although most of the changes seen with this disorder are due to the excessive secretion of cortisol, hypersecretion of other steroids may also be responsible. In bitches with Cushing's syndrome, 20 to 30% have clitoral enlargement as the result of hypersecretion of androgens. Although rare, electrolyte abnormalities are seen in some cases of Cushing's syndrome, especially those due to an adrenocortical tumor that secretes aldosterone.

Etiology

A number of different lesions or functional abnormalities can produce Cushing's syndrome in the dog. The first description of this disorder in man was written by Harvey Cushing, who described a patient that had a basophilic adenoma of the anterior pituitary, with a resulting bilateral adrenocortical hyperplasia. Based on this original description, the condition is termed Cushing's disease when the abnormality is due to a functional pituitary tumor secreting excessive ACTH. Whenever the equivalent disorder is present, but there is no pituitary tumor, it is called Cushing's syndrome. However, since occasionally it is difficult to determine the specific etiology, some clinicians call all hyperfunctional adrenocortical diseases with an excessive production of cortisol, Cushing's syndrome.

Essentially four major factors cause Cushing's syndrome. It may result from a pituitary tumor that secretes excessive ACTH. Anterior pituitary tumors producing Cushing's syndrome in the dog are usually chromophobic adenomas or adenocarcinomas, rather than basophilic tumors as described in man. Based on some studies, probably no more than 10 to 15% of all cases of canine Cushing's syndrome are due to functioning anterior pituitary tumors. Another cause of this disorder is the functional adrenocortical tumor, either an adenoma or an adenocarcinoma. Less than 5% of spontaneous cases of canine Cushing's syndrome result from functional adrenal tumors. When present, these tumors are usually unilateral.

The most common cause of Cushing's syndrome appears to be an abnormality in the negative feedback mechanism that normally controls the secretion of corticotropin-releasing factor (CRF) and ACTH. Increasing levels of cortisol, which normally inhibit CRF and ACTH production, are not effective. Excessive secretion of ACTH produces bilateral adrenocortical hyperplasia. Another cause of this disorder is the exogenous administration of steroids over a long period of time. The clinical signs and laboratory findings are essentially identical to those of spontaneous Cushing's syndrome. However, following discontinuance of the steroid administration, the iatrogenic Cushing's syndrome may take as long as one year to regress.

Pathologic Findings

Spontaneous canine Cushing's syndrome in approximately 95% of the cases is the result of hypersecretion of ACTH, whether due to a functional pituitary tumor or a defect in the negative feedback mechanism. Thus, this large percentage of cases has bilateral adrenocortical hyperplasia. The degree of hyperplasia is usually extensive, and the cortex is twice its normal size or greater (Figs.

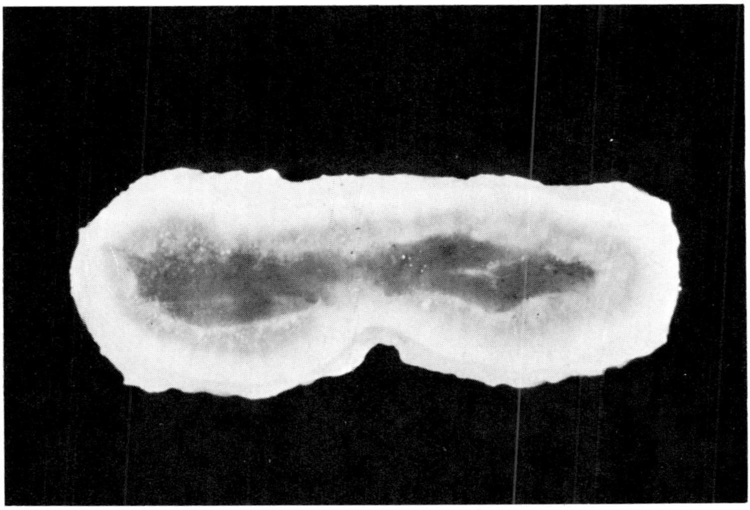

Fig. 10–7. Diffuse adrenocortical hyperplasia. Cut section of adrenal gland showing extensive adrenocortical hyperplasia. (Courtesy John T. McGrath, University of Pennsylvania.)

10–7, 10–8, and 10–9). Occasionally the adrenal glands may not be enlarged grossly, but a cut section shows that the gland is composed mainly of cortical tissue.

Approximately half of the adrenocortical tumors are adenomas (Fig. 10–10), and the other half are adenocarcinomas (Fig. 10–11). The adenocarcinomas may be both invasive and metastatic (Fig. 10–12). Some of the adenocarcinomas of the right adrenal gland invade and grow into the vena cava.

Clinical Signs

Canine Cushing's syndrome is rare before the age of five years, and is seen usually in dogs seven years of age and older. This disorder affects mainly purebred dogs, although mongrels are occasionally affected. At one time it was reported that the Boston terrier breed has a very high incidence, but more recent reports have indicated that miniature and toy poodles and dachshunds are the breeds most commonly affected.

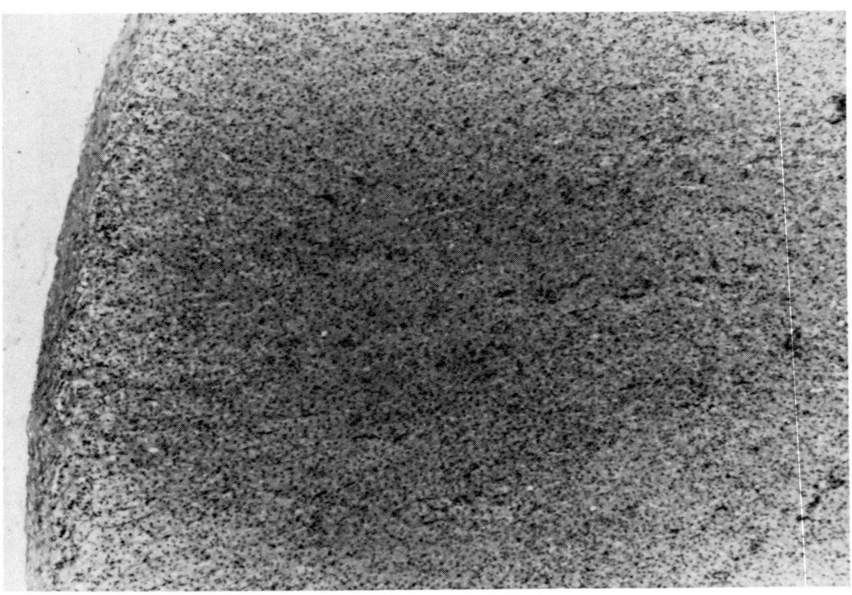

Fig. 10–8. Diffuse adrenocortical hyperplasia ×34. The hyperplastic changes affect predominately the zona fasciculata. (Courtesy John T. McGrath, University of Pennsylvania.)

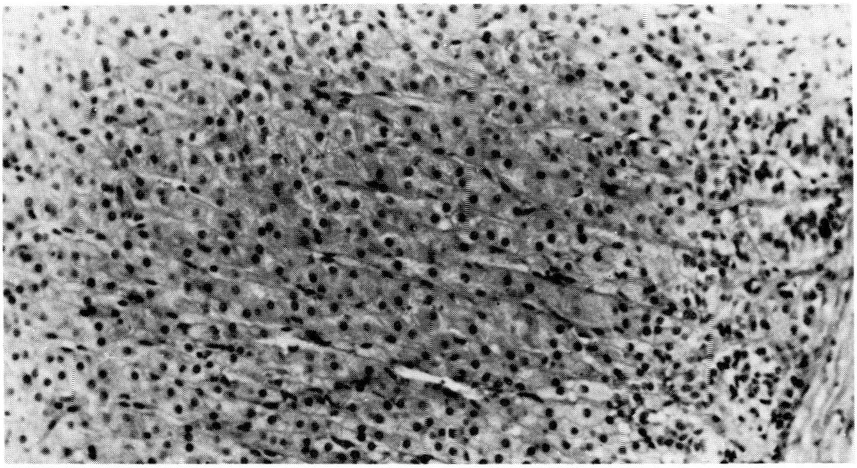

Fig. 10–9. Diffuse adrenocortical hyperplasia ×102. Higher magnification of Fig. 10–8, illustrating the alterations in the zona fasciculata. (Courtesy John T. McGrath, University of Pennsylvania.)

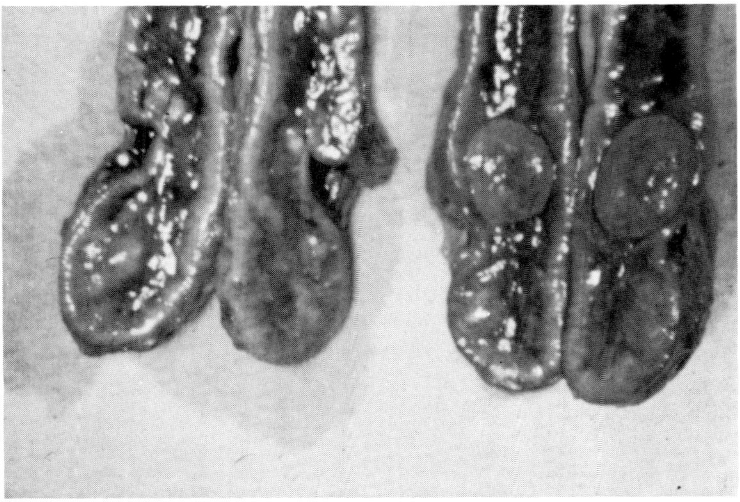

Fig. 10–10. Adrenocortical adenoma. Cut sections of adrenal glands showing a well-circumscribed adenoma in one of the glands.

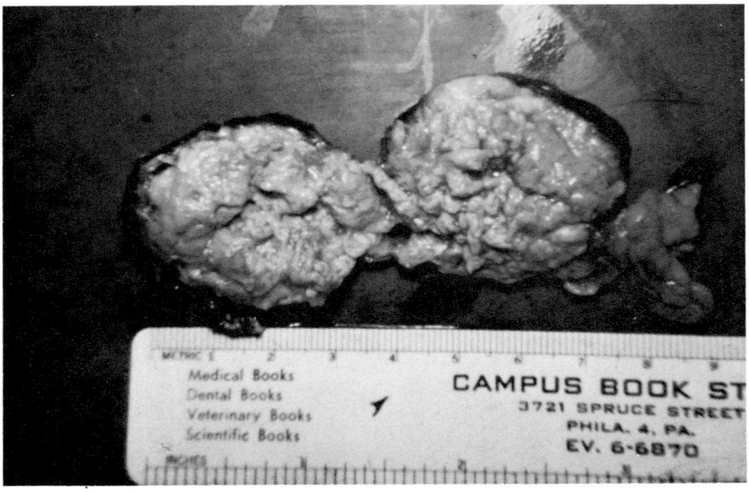

Fig. 10–11. Adrenocortical adenocarcinoma. Cut section.

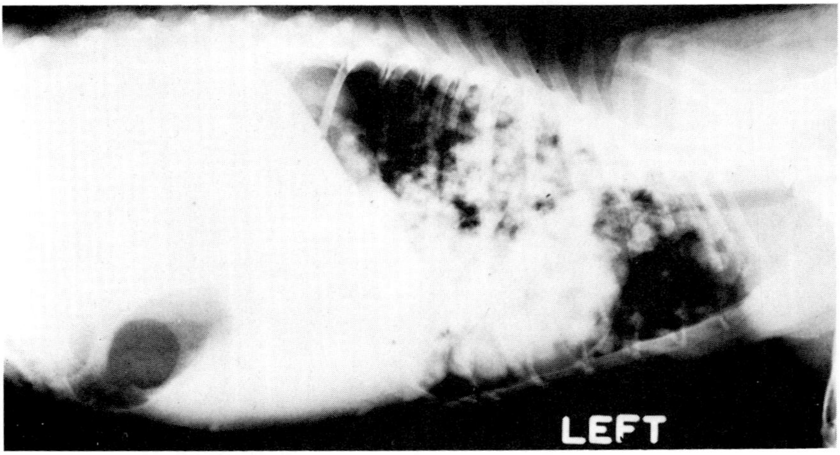

Fig. 10–12. Metastatic adrenocortical adenocarcinoma. Lateral radiograph of the chest of the dog with the tumor shown in Fig. 10–11. Extensive pulmonary metastases are present.

The first clinical signs noticed by the owner are usually polyuria, polydipsia, and a ravenous appetite. In most cases the polydipsia and polyuria are present for four to six months before the development of noticeable alopecia. The loss of hair extends over most of the body, but it rarely affects the head or the lower parts of the legs. The severity of the hair loss depends on the breed of dog. In some breeds, such as the miniature and toy poodle, Scottish terrier, Dandie Dinmont terrier, Skye terrier, and cocker spaniel, the hair loss over the body eventually becomes almost complete (Fig. 10–13). In other breeds, such as the Boston terrier, dachshund, and the giant breeds, the hair loss is less extensive. Usually it is only a thinning of the haircoat (Fig. 10–14). In those breeds that have a complete loss of hair, approximately one year elapses from the beginning of the hair loss until the alopecia is relatively complete.

The abdomen may become pendulous, producing a potbellied appearance. This condition is caused by the muscular weakness of the abdominal wall and the enlarged liver, which displaces the abdominal viscera. Anestrus is an early clinical sign that occurs in most intact females with Cushing's syndrome. In approximately 30% of the affected male dogs, testicular atrophy is seen. In 20 to 30% of female dogs, enlargement of the clitoris is evident, suggesting an excessive secretion of androgens in these cases. Occasionally well-circumscribed and delineated areas of calcinosis cutis are present.

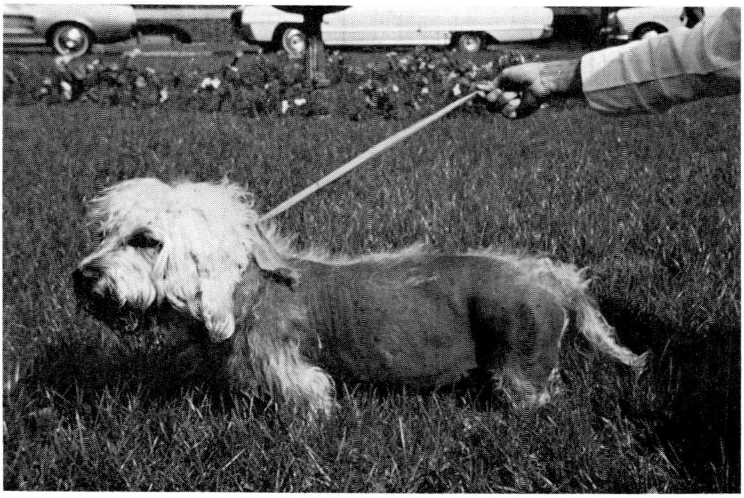

Fig. 10–13. Seven-year-old female Dandie Dinmont terrier with Cushing's syndrome. There is almost total alopecia over the body. The hair on the head and lower parts of the legs is not affected to any extent.

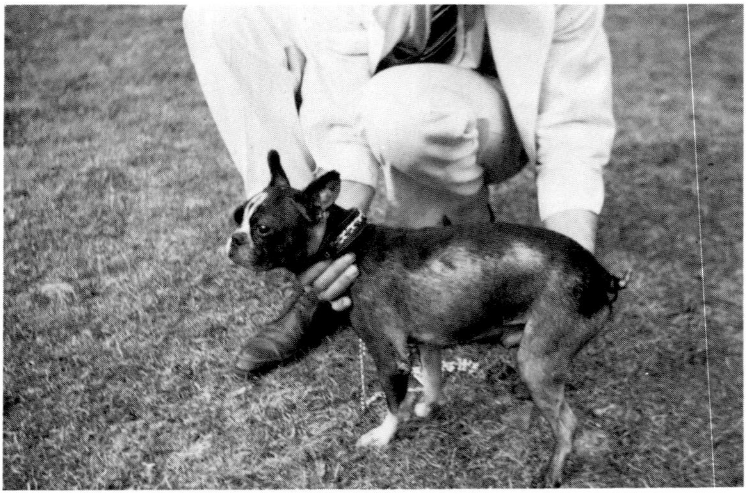

Fig. 10–14. Eight-year-old male Boston terrier with Cushing's syndrome. There is thinning of the haircoat over the body and parts of the legs.

Although calcification of the skin is not seen grossly, skin biopsy taken from most of these patients reveals histologic evidence of calcium deposition. As this disorder progresses, there is a characteristic thinning of the skin. This dermal atrophy is due to a breakdown of collagen and elastic fibers, resulting in a loss of elasticity. The skin is like that of a dehydrated animal.

Laboratory Findings

Hypercortisolism has a pronounced effect on circulating lymphocytes and eosinophils, producing a lymphopenia and eosinopenia. Usually the lymphocyte count is less than 15% on a differential white blood count, and the total eosinophil count is usually below 100/cu mm (normal is 300 to 500/cu mm). Many times the latter count is reported as zero. The serum electrolyte levels are usually normal in Cushing's syndrome, since the disorder is mainly an excess of glucocorticoids. With adrenocortical tumors accompanied by an excessive secretion of aldosterone, hypokalemia is present. Laboratory findings are consistent with the hepatic dysfunction that is present in these animals. Hypercholesterolemia and an increase in the serum alkaline phosphatase are usually seen.

For a diagnosis to be definitive, increased secretion of the corticosteroids must be demonstrated. One of the simpler techniques is to evaluate the plasma cortisol level before and after ACTH stimulation. Using 0.125 mg of synthetic ACTH (Cortrosyn) intramuscularly, it is possible to diagnose Cushing's syndrome and differentiate between a functional adrenocortical tumor and bilateral adrenocortical hyperplasia. With functional adrenocortical tumors, plasma cortisol levels are elevated, but 30 minutes following ACTH administration, there is little or no response. When bilateral adrenocortical hyperplasia is present, the preinjection plasma cortisol level may be high-normal or elevated, but characteristically there is an exaggerated response to ACTH. In the normal dog the amount of ACTH administered in this test produces a plasma cortisol response of 4 to 6 $\mu g\%$ above the preinjection level. The exaggerated response seen with bilateral adrenocortical hyperplasia usually produces plasma cortisol levels 20 to 40 $\mu g\%$ above the preinjection level.

To determine whether the bilateral adrenocortical hyperplasia is the result of a functional anterior pituitary tumor or a defect in the negative feedback mechanism requires more documentation. However, since most pituitary tumors in the dog are relatively slow growing, the presence of a pituitary tumor may not be significant, at least on a practical basis, if the abnormal adrenocortical function is corrected. Since it may take many years before the pituitary tumor causes neurologic disturbances, it may not be of utmost importance to definitely establish whether a pituitary tumor is present initially. In the rare case in which a large pituitary tumor infringes on the optic chiasm and produces a visual disturbance, or grows into the brain producing neurologic signs, it is usually not treatable.

Therapy

Different procedures have been developed for treating canine Cushing's syndrome. Unilateral adrenocortical tumors, if not metastatic, should be removed surgically. However, the contralateral adrenal is atrophied; thus, after removal of the tumorous one, the animal has to be maintained with exogenous steroids until the atrophied adrenal is functional again. At surgery the medical management is similar to that needed for bilateral adrenalectomy. Complete replacement of the corticosteroids is instituted and continued for a number of days, at the same time ACTH gel is administered intramuscularly every other day until the adrenal gland is functional again.

Two surgical techniques have been prescribed for treatment of bilateral adrenocortical hyperplasia. Bilateral adrenalectomy has been carried out by some investigators (Figs. 10–15 to 10–20), whereas others have reported clinical remissions using hypophysectomy. Both procedures have equally satisfactory results. Following bilateral adrenalectomy, it is necessary to maintain the animal on mineralocorticoid replacement therapy for life. With hypophysectomy, thyroxine therapy is needed, and occasionally a resulting diabetes insipidus

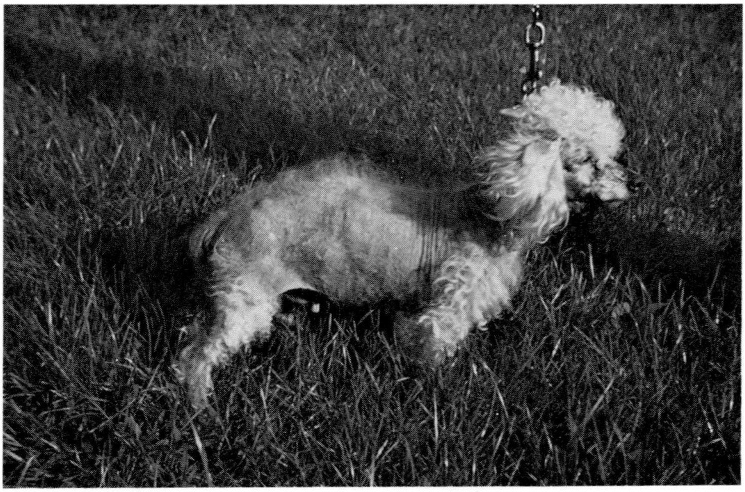

Fig. 10–15. Thirteen-year-old female toy poodle with Cushing's syndrome before bilateral adrenalectomy. (From Siegel, E. T., et al.: J. Am. Vet. Med. Assoc., *157*:2082, 1970.)

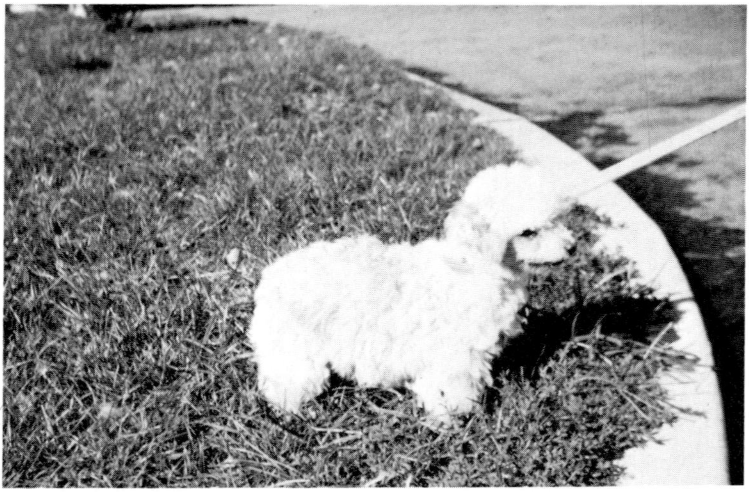

Fig. 10–16. Toy poodle shown in Fig. 10–15, eight months after bilateral adrenalectomy. (From Siegel, E. T., et al.: J. Am. Vet. Med. Assoc., *157*:2082, 1970.)

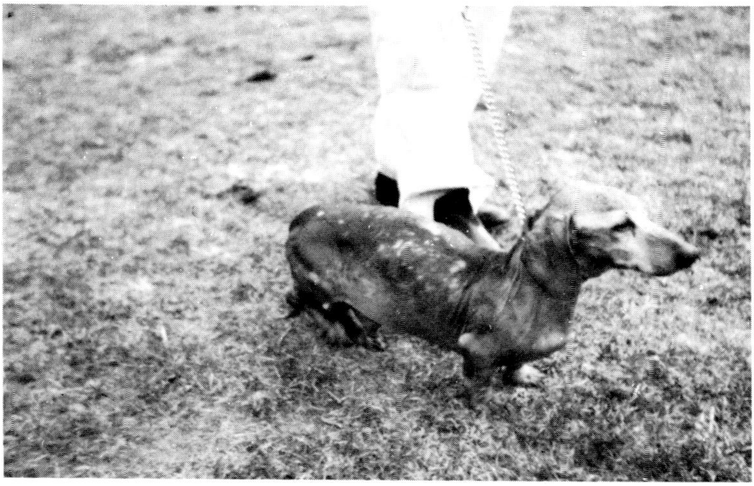

Fig. 10–17. Dachshund (5½ years old) with Cushing's syndrome before bilateral adrenalectomy. (From Siegel, E. T., et al.: J. Am. Vet. Med. Assoc., *157*:2084, 1970.)

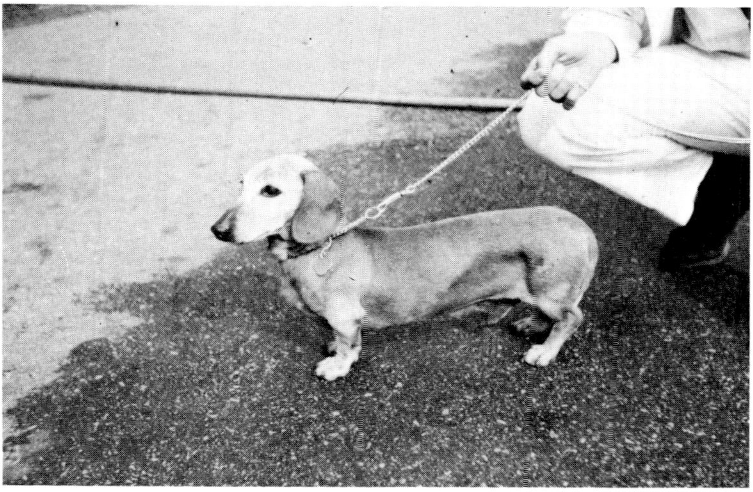

Fig. 10–18. Dachshund shown in Fig. 10–17, six months after bilateral adrenalectomy. (From Siegel, E. T., et al.: J. Am. Vet. Med. Assoc., *157*:2084, 1970.)

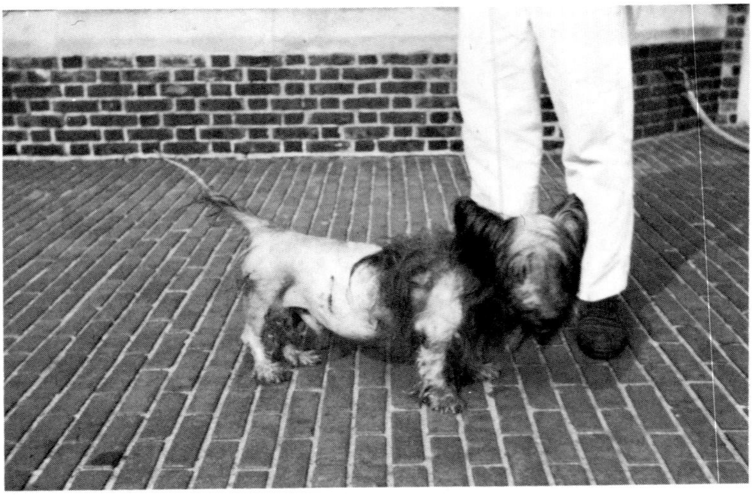

Fig. 10–19. Eight-year-old male Skye terrier with Cushing's syndrome one week after bilateral adrenalectomy. (From Siegel, E. T., et al.: J. Am. Vet. Med. Assoc., *157*:2083, 1970.)

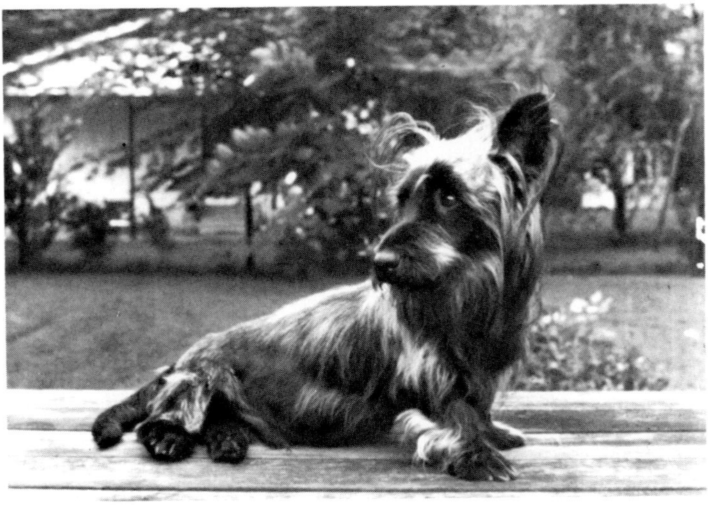

Fig. 10–20. Skye terrier shown in Fig. 10–19, seven months after bilateral adrenalectomy. (From Siegel, E. T., et al.: J. Am. Vet. Med. Assoc., *157*:2083, 1970.)

needs treatment with intramuscular injections of vasopressin tannate in oil. Pituitary irradiation is successful in man, but this technique has not been utilized in dogs with Cushing's syndrome.

In performing a bilateral adrenalectomy, preoperative steroid therapy is started two days before surgery. One to two mg of desoxycorticosterone acetate (DOCA) is administered s.i.d. (once a day) and 25 to 50 mg of cortisone acetate b.i.d. (twice a day) intramuscularly. This treatment is continued through the morning of surgery. Cortisol hemisuccinate (100 mg) in saline solution with dextrose is infused during surgery. The cortisol hemisuccinate solution is dripped slowly until the blood vessels of the second adrenal are being ligated. At that time the flow is increased. Another 100-mg infusion of cortisol hemisuccinate is given later on the first day of surgery. Following surgery, the DOCA dosage is adjusted until the serum sodium and potassium levels are stabilized in the normal range. Cortisone acetate administration is continued, but 48 hours after surgery the dosage is decreased gradually, so that the amount of glucocorticoid is completely withdrawn within seven to ten days after surgery. Then DOCA pellets can be implanted for long-term therapy control. Salt is administered in the food daily, and cortisol tablets (5 mg) may be administered per os for stress.

Recent reports have described use of the adrenotoxic compound, o,p'-DDD, 1, 1 dichloro-2(o-chlorophenyl)-2-(p-chlorophenyl) ethane, for treatment of Cushing's syndrome in the dog. DDD, an analog of DDT, was first produced commercially as an insecticide. Early toxicologic studies revealed that DDD produced adrenocortical necrosis and atrophy in dogs. Later findings showed that one of the isomers present in the mixture of DDD, o,p'-DDD, was responsible for the hemorrhagic necrosis of the canine adrenal cortex. The cytotoxic action of o,p'-DDD is not completely understood. In addition to the destruction of the cortical tissue, o,p'-DDD has an effect on extra-adrenal steroid metabolism and degradation, in particular an alteration of the cortisol metabolism. This change, which seems to occur mainly from the induction of a 6β-hydroxylase in the liver, results in the formation of 6β-hydroxycortisol. This catabolite of cortisol has minimal solubility in the commonly used organic solvents for measurement of urinary excretion of 17-hydroxycorticosteroids. Therefore, if a urinary 17-hydroxycorticosteroid method is used to monitor a response to o,p'-DDD, the values obtained may give a misleading suggestion that production of these compounds has decreased. A better method of evaluating the effect of o,p'-DDD is to assay the direct levels of cortisol or the cortisol secretion rate.

One difficulty with the use of o,p'-DDD in the treatment of Cushing's syndrome is that the effective dose for therapy and the systemic toxic dose are sometimes nearly identical. Using the drug conservatively, only a temporary regression may occur. Although clinical signs may ameliorate, in time Cushing's syndrome recurs. If large doses of o,p′-DDD are given, an acute adrenocortical insufficiency may be produced. Although o,p′-DDD primarily affects the zona reticularis and fasciculata, sparing the zona glomerulosa, large doses of the drug produce acute adrenal insufficiency. One possible therapeutic procedure is the deliberate production of adrenal insufficiency while the animal is on replacement therapy.

The most compelling reason for not using o,p′-DDD is the high incidence of mortality reported. In two different studies, approximately one out of three dogs so treated died suddenly while being medicated with o,p′-DDD. What seems to be a 30% mortality rate with this drug is not acceptable when compared to the 90 to 95% success rate reported with bilateral adrenalectomy. The high toxicity of o,p′-DDD is the reason for discontinuing its use in treatment of Cushing's syndrome in man. Presently o,p′-DDD is recommended only for those persons with inoperable metastatic adrenocortical carcinoma. I believe that o,p′-DDD in therapy in the dog should also be restricted to those cases that are not correctable by surgery.

Other Adrenal Disorders

Aldosteronism, congenital adrenal hyperplasia (adrenogenital syndrome), and adrenal feminization have not been described in the dog. Hypersecretion of aldosterone in man produces hypertension and hypokalemia. Congenital adrenal hyperplasia results from the insufficiency or absence of one of three important adrenal enzymes necessary in the biosynthesis of cortisol. This enzyme defect produces a decrease in the negative feedback control of ACTH. The resultant increase in ACTH secretion stimulates the adrenal gland and the biosynthesis up to the enzyme block. An increase in some of the intermediate metabolites of cortisol occurs, and these metabolites are then converted to androgens. Adrenal feminization, a rare disorder in man, is associated with undifferentiated neoplastic tumors.

Adrenal medullary insufficiency is not recognizable clinically. In contrast, hypersecretion of catecholamines occurs associated with adrenal medullary tumors, pheochromocytomas. Such tumors have been seen in the dog. It is rare for clinical signs to occur with these tumors unless they are invasive and affect other vital organs. The pheochromocytoma in man is notorious for secreting both epinephrine and norepinephrine, thus producing hypertension. Since blood pressure readings are not a routine procedure in the dog, pheochromocytomas are rarely diagnosed.

SELECTED READING

1. Annis, J. R.: Adrenal cortical failure in the dog. Vet. Med., *55*:35, 1960
2. Azuma, T., and Eisenstein, A. B.: Effect of adrenal steroids on carbohydrate metabolism in various animal species. Endocrinology, *75*:521, 1964.
3. Balazs, T.: Effects of DDD and DDT on the production and metabolism of adrenocortical steroids in guinea pigs and dogs. Am. J. Vet. Res., *30*:1535, 1969.
4. Baxter, J. D., and Forsham, P. H.: Tissue effects of glucocorticoids. Am. J. Med., *53*:573, 1972.
5. Baylink, D. J., and Hurxthal, L. M.: Assessment of adrenocortical function. Postgrad. Med., *33*:20, 1963.
6. Beierwaltes, W. H., et al.: Imaging functional nodules of the adrenal glands with ^{131}I-19-iodocholesterol. J. Nucl. Med., *15*:246, 1974.
7. Beisel, W. R., and Rapoport, M. I.: Inter-relations between adrenocortical functions and infectious illness. N. Engl. J. Med., *280*:541, 1969.
8. Bethge, H., Bayer, J. M., and Winkelmann, W.: Diagnosis of Cushing's syndrome. Acta Endocrinol., *60*:47, 1969.
9. Biglieri, E. G.: Hypertension with primary and secondary hyperaldosteronism. Postgrad. Med., *52*:78, 1972.
10. Blair, R. J., et al.: Radiolabeled cholesterol as an adrenal scanning agent. J. Nucl. Med., *12*:176, 1971.
11. Blizzard, R. M., et al.: Adrenal antibodies in Addison's disease. Lancet *2*:901, 1962.
12. Bongiovanni, A. M.: Fluid therapy in adrenocortical failure. Pediatr. Clin. North Am., *11*:971, 1964.
13. Bozzini, C. E., Rendo, M. E. B., and Kofoed, J. A.: Erythrokinetics in adrenalectomized dogs. Acta Physiol. Lat. Am., *18*:304, 1968.
14. Bransome, E. D., Jr.: Adrenal cortex. Annu. Rev. Physiol., *30*:171, 1968.
15. Brownie, A. C., and Sprunt, J. G.: Metopirone in the assessment of pituitary-adrenal function. Lancet, *1*:773, 1962.
16. Bush, I. E.: Chemical and biological factors in the activity of adrenocortical steroids. Pharmacol. Rev., *14*:317, 1962.
17. Carey, L. C., and Ellison, E. H.: Adrenalectomy: technique, errors, and pitfalls. Surg. Clin. North Am., *46*:1283, 1966.
18. Carney, J. A., Sizemore, G. W., and Tyce, G. M.: Bilateral adrenal medullary hyperplasia in multiple endocrine neoplasia, type 2. The precursor of bilateral pheochromocytoma. Mayo Clin. Proc., *50*:3, 1975.
19. Coffin, D. L., and Munson, T. O.: Endocrine diseases of the dog associated with hair loss. J. Am. Vet. Med. Assoc., *123*:402, 1953.
20. Collins, E. J., Carpenter, O. S., and Baker, V. F.: Influence of adrenal steroids on radio-calcium metabolism in young beagle dogs. Acta Endocrinol., *42*:348, 1963.
21. Collins, E. J., Garrett, E. R., and Johnston, R. L.: Effect of adrenal steroids on radio-calcium metabolism in dogs. Metabolism, *11*:716, 1962.
22. Croughs, R. J. M., Tops, C. F., and De Jong, F. H.: Radioimmunoassay of plasma adrenocorticotrophin in Cushing's syndrome. J. Endocrinol., *59*:439, 1973.
23. Dluhy, R. G., Himathongkam, T., and Greenfield, M.: Rapid ACTH test with plasma aldosterone levels. Ann. Intern. Med., *80*:693, 1974.
24. Dorfman, R. I.: Symposium: adrenal steroids. A system of evaluating the functional status of the adrenal cortex. Metabolism, *10*:902, 1961.
25. Ehrlich, E. N.: Aldosterone, the adrenal cortex, and hypertension. Annu. Rev. Med., *19*:373, 1968.
26. Eisenstein, A. B.: Addison's disease: etiology and relationship to other endocrine disorders. Med. Clin. North Am., *52*:327, 1968.
27. Fukuda, T., and Koyama, T.: On the significance of acidosis in adrenal insufficiency Jap. J. Physiol., *12*:176, 1962.
28. Gitlow, S. E., Pertsemlidis, D., and Bertani, L. M.: Management of patients with pheochromocytoma. Am. Heart J., *82*:557, 1971.
29. Gordon, E. S.: Importance of adrenal gland in diagnosis and treatment of hypertension. Postgrad. Med., *40*:138, 1966.
30. Hoffman, D. L., and Mattox, V. R.: Treatment of adrenocortical carcinoma with o,p'-DDD. Med. Clin. North Am., *56*:999, 1972.

31. Howard, E. B., and Nielsen, S. W.: Pheochromocytomas associated with hypertensive lesions in dogs. J. Am. Vet. Med. Assoc., *147*:245, 1965.
32. Hughes, S. W. M., and Burley, D. M.: Aminoglutethimide: a "side-effect" turned to therapeutic advantage. Postgrad. Med. J., *46*:409, 1970.
33. Jacobson, M. E.: The rationale of alternate-day corticosteroid therapy. Clin. Pharmacol., *49*:181, 1971.
34. Kahn, P. C.: The radiologic identification of functioning adrenal tumors. Radiol. Clin. North Am., *5*:221, 1967.
35. Kappas, A., and Palmer, R. H.: Selected aspects of steroid pharmacology. Pharmacol. Rev., *15*:123, 1963.
36. Kelly, D. F.: Necrosis of the adrenal cortex and adrenal capsular myoarteritis in a dog. Vet. Rec., *77*:998, 1965.
37. Kennedy, J. H., Williams, M. J., and Sommers, S. C.: Cushing's syndrome and cancer of the lung: pituitary Crooke cell hyperplasia in pulmonary oat cell carcinoma. Ann. Surg., *160*:90, 1964.
38. Liddle, G. W.: Analysis of circadian rhythms in human adrenocortical secretory activity. Arch. Intern. Med., *117*:739, 1966.
39. Lorenz, M. D., and Scott, D. W.: Treatment of canine Cushing's disease with o,p′-DDD: a summary. J. Am. Anim. Hosp. Assoc., *8*:388, 1972.
40. Lorenz, M. D., Scott, D. W., and Pulley, L. T.: Medical treatment of canine hyperadrenocorticoidism with o,p′-DDD. Cornell Vet., *63*:646, 1973.
41. Marshak, R. R., Webster, G. D., and Skelley, J. F.: Adrenocortical insufficiency in a dog. J. Am. Vet. Med. Assoc., *136*:274, 1960.
42. Martin, J. E., Skillen, R. G., and Deubler, M. J.: The action of adrenocorticotropic hormone on circulating eosinophils in dogs — a proposed screening method for evaluating adrenal cortical function. Am. J. Vet. Res., *15*:489, 1954.
43. Mathur, R. S., et al.: In vitro sterol and steroid biogenesis by a feminizing adrenocortical carcinoma. Acta Endocrinol., *73*:518, 1973.
44. McGiff, J. C.: Tissue hormones: angiotensin, bradykinin and the regulation of regional blood flows. Med. Clin. North Am., *52*:263, 1968.
45. McManus, J. L., Nimmons, C. B., and Buchta, W.: Surgical and medical management of hyperadrenocorticalism in a Boston terrier. Can. Vet. J., *11*:78, 1970.
46. Moorhead, E. L., et al.: The diagnosis of pheochromocytoma. J.A.M.A., *196*:1107, 1966.
47. Murison, P. J.: Hyperfunctioning adrenocortical diseases. Med. Clin. North Am., *51*:883, 1967.
48. Nattrass, M., et al.: Plasma-corticosteroid determinations for assessment of pituitary response to metyrapone. Lancet, *2*:903, 1972.
49. Nelson, D. H.: Relative merits of the adrenocortical steroids. Annu. Rev. Med., *13*:241, 1962.
50. Nelson, D. H.: Regulation of glucocorticoid release. Am. J. Med., *53*:590, 1972.
51. New, M. I.: Congenital adrenal hyperplasia. Pediatr. Clin. North Am., *15*:395, 1968.
52. O'Neal, L. W.: Pathologic anatomy in Cushing's syndrome. Ann. Surg., *160*:860, 1964.
53. Reece, W. O.: Fluid volume changes associated with withdrawal and restoration of steroid therapy in adrenalectomized dogs. Am. J. Vet. Res., *33*:1493, 1972.
54. Reidenberg, M. M., et al.: Hemodynamic changes in adrenalectomized dogs. Endocrinology, *72*:918, 1963.
55. Rhamy, R. K., et al.: Primary aldosteronism: experience with current diagnostic criteria and surgical treatment in fourteen patients. Ann. Surg., *167*:718, 1968.
56. Rijnberk, A., Der Kinderen, P. J., and Thijssen, J. H. H.: Spontaneous hyperadrenocorticism in the dog. J. Endocrinol., *41*:397, 1968.
57. Rossi, P.: Arteriography in adrenal tumours. Br. J. Radiol., *41*:81, 1968.
58. Rothenbacher, H., and Shigley, R. F.: Adrenocortical apoplexy in a dog. J. Am. Vet. Med. Assoc., *149*:406, 1966.
59. Sachs, B. A.: Endocrine disorders produced by nonendocrine malignant tumors. Bull. N. Y. Acad. Med., *41*:1069, 1965.

60. Sanzari, N. P., Possanza, G., and Troop, R. C.: Lack of correlation between body weight and cortisol secretion, and between adrenal weight and cortisol secretion in the dog. Life Sci., *4*:1345, 1965.
61. Schambelan, M., Stockigt, J. R., and Biglieri, E. G.: Isolated hypoaldosteronism in adults. N. Engl. J. Med., *287*:573, 1972.
62. Schechter, R. D., et al.: Treatment of Cushing's syndrome in the dog with an adrenocorticolytic agent (o,p'DDD). J. Am. Vet. Med. Assoc., *162*:629, 1973.
63. Scheiner, E., Isaacs, M., and Vanamee, P.: Water and electrolyte disturbances in cancer patients. Med. Clin. North Am., *50*:711, 1966.
64. Segre, E. J., et al.: Hirsutism and virilizing syndromes. Annu. Rev. Med., *15*:315, 1964.
65. Siegel, E. T.: Determination of 17-hydroxycorticosteroids in canine urine. Am. J. Vet. Res., *26*:1152, 1965.
66. Siegel, E. T., et al.: Functional adrenocortical carcinoma in a dog. J. Am. Vet. Med. Assoc., *150*:760, 1967.
67. Sih, C. J., and Whitlock, H. W., Jr.: Biochemistry of steroids. Annu. Rev. Biochem., *37*:661, 1968.
68. Singer, M. M.: Endocrine emergencies: Med. Clin. North Am., *55*:1315, 1971.
69. Speckart, P. F., Nicoloff, J. T., and Bethune, J. E.: Screening for adrenocortical insufficiency with cosyntropin (synthetic ACTH). Arch. Intern. Med., *128*:761, 1971.
70. Strauch, G. O., and Vinnick, L.: Persistent Cushing's syndrome apparently cured by ectopic adrenalectomy. J.A.M.A., *221*:183, 1972.
71. Swingle, W. W., and Swingle, A. J.: Effect of adrenal steroids upon plasma volume of intact and adrenalectomized dogs. Proc. Soc. Exp. Biol. Med., *119*:452, 1965.
72. Swingle, W. W., and Swingle, A. J.: Terminal insufficiency in adrenalectomized dogs maintained for three years on substitution therapy and the apparent absence of accessory cortical tissue in this species. Endocrinology, *81*:406, 1967.
73. Temple, T. E., Jr., et al.: Treatment of Cushing's disease. N. Engl. J. Med., *281*:801, 1969.
74. Temple, T. E., Jr., and Liddle, G. W.: Inhibitors of adrenal steroid biosynthesis. Annu. Rev. Pharmacol., *10*:199, 1970.
75. Thorn, G. W.: The adrenal cortex. Johns Hopkins Med. J., *123*:49, 1968.
76. Tucci, J. R., et al.: Rapid dexamethasone suppression test for Cushing's syndrome. J.A.M.A., *199*:379, 1967.
77. Tyler, F. H., and West, C. D.: Laboratory evaluation of disorders of the adrenal cortex. Am. J. Med., *53*:664, 1972.
78. Vagnucci, A. H.: Selective aldosterone deficiency. J. Clin. Endocrinol. Metab., *29*:279, 1969.
79. Venning, E. H.: Adenohypophysis and adrenal cortex. Annu. Rev. Physiol., *27*:107, 1965.
80. Walser, M., Robinson, B. H. B., and Duckett, J. W.: The hypercalcemia of adrenal insufficiency. J. Clin. Invest., *42*:456, 1963.
81. Wegienka, L. C., Grasso, S. G., and Forsham, P. H.: Estimation of adrenomedullary reserve by infusion of 2-deoxy-D-glucose. J. Clin. Endocrinol. Metab., *26*:37, 1966.
82. Werk, E. E., Jr., Sholiton, L. J., and Kalejs, L.: Testosterone-secreting adrenal adenoma under gonadotropin control. N. Engl. J. Med., *289*:767, 1973.
83. Wilson, R. B., et al.: Response of dogs to corticotropin measured by 17-hydroxycorticosteroid excretion. Am. J. Vet. Res., *28*:313, 1967.
84. Zimmermann, B.: Pituitary and adrenal function in relation to surgery. Surg. Clin. North Am., *45*:299, 1965.

Chapter

11

The Gonads

In this era of sensitive hormonal assays, surprisingly little information is available on the normal levels of hormones in the dog. More than any other factor, the cost of some of the assay procedures probably has hampered the development of knowledge in this area. In man, gonadotropin, estrogen, and progesterone assays are routinely used in the evaluation of endocrinologic disorders in the female. In the dog some of the basic information on hormonal levels has not yet been confirmed.

Because of the lack of specific information on the canine gonad, this area of study is plagued by rather crude clinical impressions or outright "wives tales." The diagnosis of hypoestrogenism in the bitch with hair loss is still made by some veterinarians, although it is well established that adrenalectomized and ovariectomized dogs maintained only on mineralocorticoids have haircoats that are normal in texture and appearance. This finding supports the conclusion that estrogens, or any other sex steroids, are not necessary for normal haircoat function in the dog. The original misinterpretation that hypoestrogenism caused hair loss probably resulted from the observation that dogs with hypercortisolism (Cushing's syndrome) were anestrous and also had hair loss. In past years Cushing's syndrome was not recognized as an adrenal disorder, so anestrus in these dogs could have been misconstrued as contributing to the development of alopecia. Although extrapolation of data from other species is often used in assessing the dog, the assumptions made may be misleading. Certain aspects of hormone secretion and catabolism can be species specific.

ESTROUS CYCLE

The dog has a monestrous cycle since one period of receptivity occurs per breeding season. Some have characterized the dog as being seasonally monestrous with specific breeding times during the year. Although some breeds of dogs more commonly come into estrus in the winter or early spring, many other breeds experience an equal distribution of the estrual cycle throughout the calendar year. The seasonal influence on the breeding season probably has become modified as the dog has become more domesticated.

Primary ovarian follicles are present in the ovary of the immature bitch as early as 15 days of age, although most of the follicles degenerate until puberty. In most dogs puberty begins between six and nine months, although some larger breeds may not reach puberty until two years of age. At that time maturing graafian follicles are present.

Usually the canine estrous cycle is divided into four stages: proestrus, estrus, metestrus, and anestrus. Proestrus is the period of follicular maturation. During this time the genital tract is being prepared for reception of the ova. The vulva swells, and the vagina discharges a bloody fluid. Proestrus normally lasts nine to ten days, but may be as short as three or as long as 16 days. During this period the vaginal smear contains many red blood cells, and there is increasing cornification of the vaginal epithelial cells. Present thought considers proestrus a period characterized by increasing levels of FSH secretion, which affect the development and maturation of the follicles. Estrogens secreted by the developing follicle affect the vaginal mucosa and receptivity. Toward the end of proestrus the bitch becomes sexually attractive to male dogs.

During estrus the bitch continues to be attractive to male dogs, and at this time she is receptive to breeding. Estrus is usually seven to nine days in length, but it may be as short as four days or as long as two weeks. During this period the follicles are large and well developed, and ovulation occurs spontaneously usually between the second and third day of estrus. Some studies suggest that ovulation in the bitch continues over a period of 12 to 72 hours. However, other studies have concluded that all of the follicles rupture simultaneously. The ova are viable for not less than 24 hours, and may be viable as long as four days. The vaginal fluid is characterized by a predominance of cornified epithelial cells and a complete absence of noncornified cells. During early estrus leukocytes are absent from the vaginal fluid; they reappear shortly after ovulation. Usually a small number of red blood cells is seen in the estrual vaginal fluid.

Metestrus has classically been defined as the "luteal phase" of the estrous cycle in the dog. However, some investigators have preferred to further divide metestrus into two different phases, metestrus being that time from ovulation until the corpora lutea become functional (approximately two days), and diestrus being that part of the cycle when progesterone is the predominant secretion of the corpora lutea. I prefer to use the classical definition of metestrus, i.e., the part of the cycle in which the corpora lutea remain functional. During metestrus the bitch rapidly loses her attractiveness to male dogs. In the nonpregnant dog, the corpora lutea begin to regress between 20 and 30 days of metestrus. In the pregnant dog, the morphology of the corpora lutea is maintained until the end of gestation. Atrophy of endometrial glands begins about the twentieth day of metestrus, but complete endometrial regression to an anestrous stage may require 80 to 90 days. Pseudocyesis is a normal stage in the dog, with most bitches showing slight mammary development six to ten weeks following estrus. Only the dogs that show exaggerated signs of pseudopregnancy attract clinical attention.

Leukocytes rapidly increase in number in the vaginal secretions during metestrus. A decrease in the percentage of cornified epithelial cells matches an increase in noncornified epithelial cells. Later during metestrus the vaginal smear consists of noncornified epithelial cells and leukocytes.

Anestrus is the quiescent period between estrual cycles. Whereas proestrus, estrus, and metestrus are fairly constant in time for different breeds of dogs, anestrus is variable. In dogs that have three estrous cycles yearly, the relative length of anestrus is shortened. During anestrus the vulva is at its smallest size, and only noncornified epithelial cells and leukocytes are seen in the vaginal smear.

During pregnancy it takes between five and ten days for the fertilized ova to reach the anterior horn of the uterus, with the embryo being in the 16- to 32-cell stage. Implantation occurs 18 to 20 days after conception, with the zonary placentas becoming established at the beginning of the second trimester of gestation. The morphology and the function of the corpora lutea are maintained until the end of gestation. Hypophysectomy at any stage of gestation in the dog results in abortion. However, ovariectomy carried out during the last half of gestation does not cause abortion.

HORMONE LEVELS IN THE BITCH

The dog excretes low levels of gonadotropins into the urine; therefore, measurement of urinary gonadotropins during the estrous cycle or pregnancy is not very revealing. It is believed that FSH is secreted during late anestrus and early proestrus, although no definitive studies have reported actual FSH levels in the dog. Serum LH has a peak concentration (27 ± 5.2 ng/ml) one day prior to standing estrus (Fig. 11–1). Estrogen levels increase during proestrus and estrus, although it appears that the dog secretes relatively small

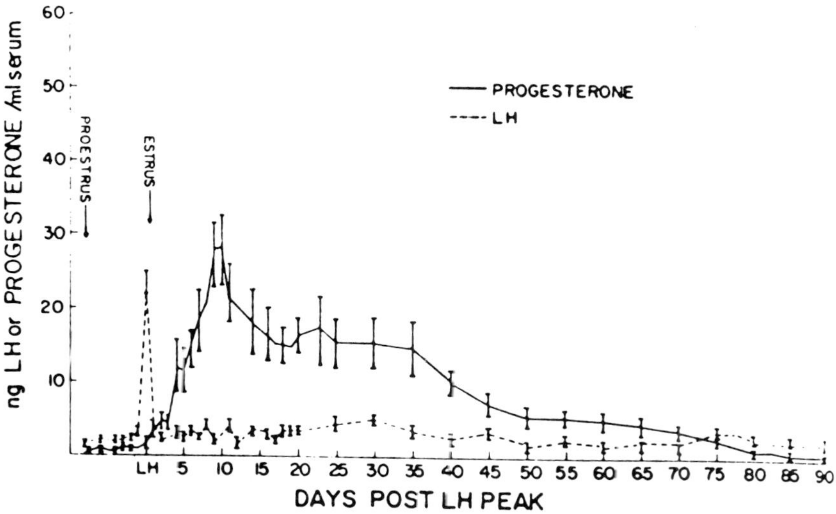

Fig. 11–1. LH and progesterone concentrations in six nonmated female dogs throughout the periods of proestrus, estrus, and corpus luteum function. Vertical bars represent the standard error of the mean. (From Smith, M. S., and McDonald, L. E.: Endocrinology, *94*:404, 1974.)

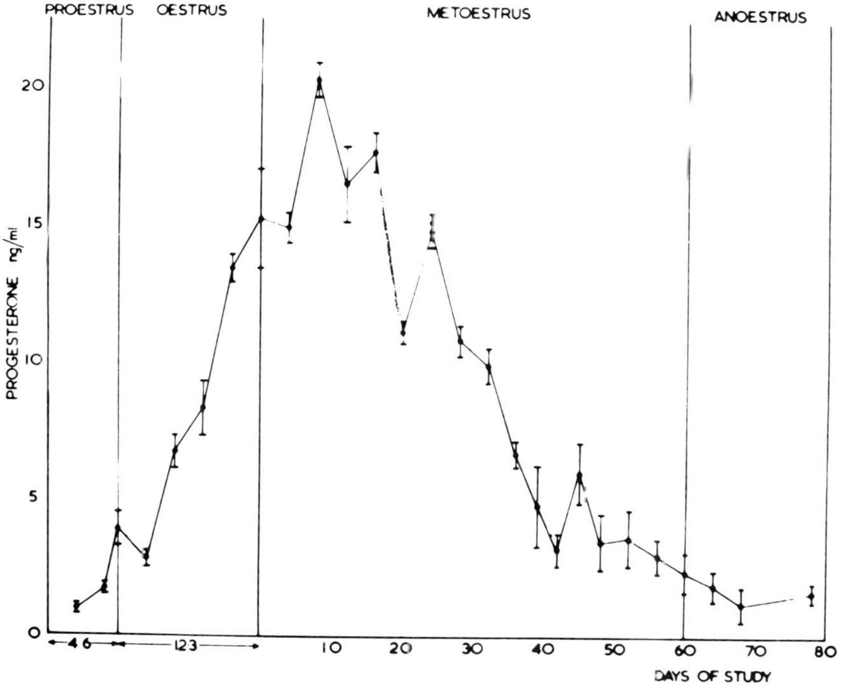

Fig. 11–2. Plasma progesterone levels during the normal estrous cycle. Mean and standard deviation of mean for 13 bitches. (From Christie, D. W., et al.: Acta Endocrinol., *68*:543, 1971.)

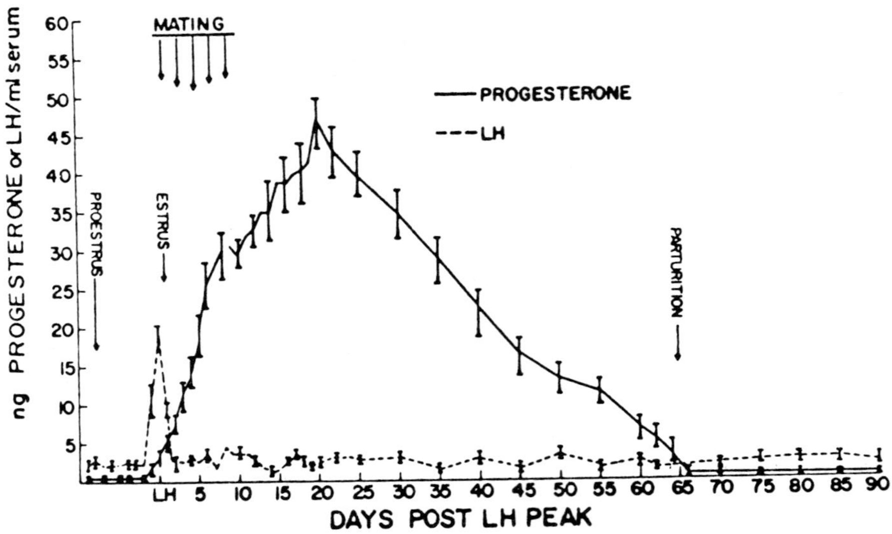

Fig. 11–3. LH and progesterone concentrations during pregnancy in nine female dogs. Vertical bars represent the standard error of the mean. (From Smith, M. S., and McDonald, L. E.: Endocrinology, *94*:404, 1974.)

amounts of estrogens throughout the estrous cycle. Serum progesterone levels rise during estrus and reach a maximum in early metestrus (Fig. 11–2). There is a great variation between dogs in respect to the magnitude and the timing of the progesterone peak. It has been reported that progesterone values reach their maximum from three days before the end of estrus to day 21 of metestrus.

In the nonpregnant bitch the level of progesterone decreases from its peak to nondetectable levels by approximately 80 days after the LH peak. However, in pregnant dogs progesterone levels generally decrease 10 to 15 days following the LH peak, but then increase to maximal levels (47 ± 3.1 ng/ml) between 20 and 25 days after the LH peak. The serum progesterone generally decreases to nondetectable levels by the day following parturition (Fig. 11–3).

ANESTRUS

Anestrus may be primary, i.e., estrus has never occurred by the time the bitch is two years of age, or it may be secondary, i.e., estrus ceases for a number of months after normal estrous cycles have been established.

With primary anestrus it should be established that the bitch is a genetic female with normal ovarian and genital development. It is worthwhile to have chromosome analysis of valuable breeding animals with anestrus. If no chromosomal abnormality exists, the noncycling bitch can be stimulated with exogenous gonadotropins. If the bitch is responsive to this therapy, fertility is often low in the induced cycle, but the animal will usually recycle without further treatment in five to eight months. Administration of pregnant mare serum (50 U/lb of body weight), up to a maximum of 1500 IU administered weekly for up to three treatments, has been successful in stimulating an induced estrus in the bitch with primary anestrus.

Secondary anestrus may result from hypothalamic, nutritional, pituitary, thyroidal, adrenal, or ovarian dysfunction. Nutritional causes of anestrus are rare, except in the extreme case of malnutrition. The inability to quantitate gonadotropin secretion routinely in the dog makes assessing hypothalamic or pituitary dysfunction impractical clinically. Anestrus is not usually seen with hypothyroidism; more commonly there is decreased fertility. The hypothyroid bitch often is less attractive to male dogs and may not accept the male readily. Anestrus is a relatively consistent finding in dogs with hypercortisolism or Cushing's syndrome. In most instances anestrus occurs early in the course of the disease, but following adrenalectomy, the normal estrous cycle recurs within one to three months.

ENDOMETRIAL CYSTIC HYPERPLASIA-PYOMETRA

Controversy has developed over the cause of endometrial cystic hyperplasia or pyometra in the bitch. Some have suggested that this disorder results from excessive stimulation of the canine uterus by progestational compounds. They reason that the disorder occurs during the progestational stage of the estrous cycle. In addition, endometrial cystic hyperplasia and pyometra have been produced by the administration of exogenous progestational compounds. Other studies have suggested that this disorder is an infectious disease resulting from certain organisms in the genital tract that may have greater infectivity during progestational stimulation. The findings by a number of clinicians of sterile uterine contents in many cases do not support the theory that infection is an essential component of this disease.

Excessive uterine stimulation by estrogens has also been suggested as the cause of this disorder. Since pyometra occurs during the part of the cycle when estrogen levels are minimal, this explanation does not seem probable. Also, if excessive estrogens are secreted during the development of this disorder, estrual signs, such as attraction of male dogs, would be seen.

Although administration of exogenous progestational compounds can produce the disease, spontaneous endometrial cystic hyperplasia-pyometra is more difficult to explain. A recent report concluded that both progesterone and estrogen levels are normal in established cases of pyometra. The author of this latter study believes that pyometra may result from defective metabolism of the hormones by the target tissue, the uterus. However, no data prove that this type of mechanism exists in the spontaneous disease. At present the cause of endometrial cystic hyperplasia-pyometra complex in the bitch is unknown, but the disease can definitely be induced by the administration of exogenous progestogens.

FUNCTIONAL OVARIAN TUMORS

The ovary is capable of synthesizing estrogens, androgens, and progestogens. The follicle is the major source of estrogen during the early part of the estrous cycle, and it can also produce androgen and progesterone. Following ovulation, the follicle is rapidly converted into a corpus luteum, which produces most of the progesterone during

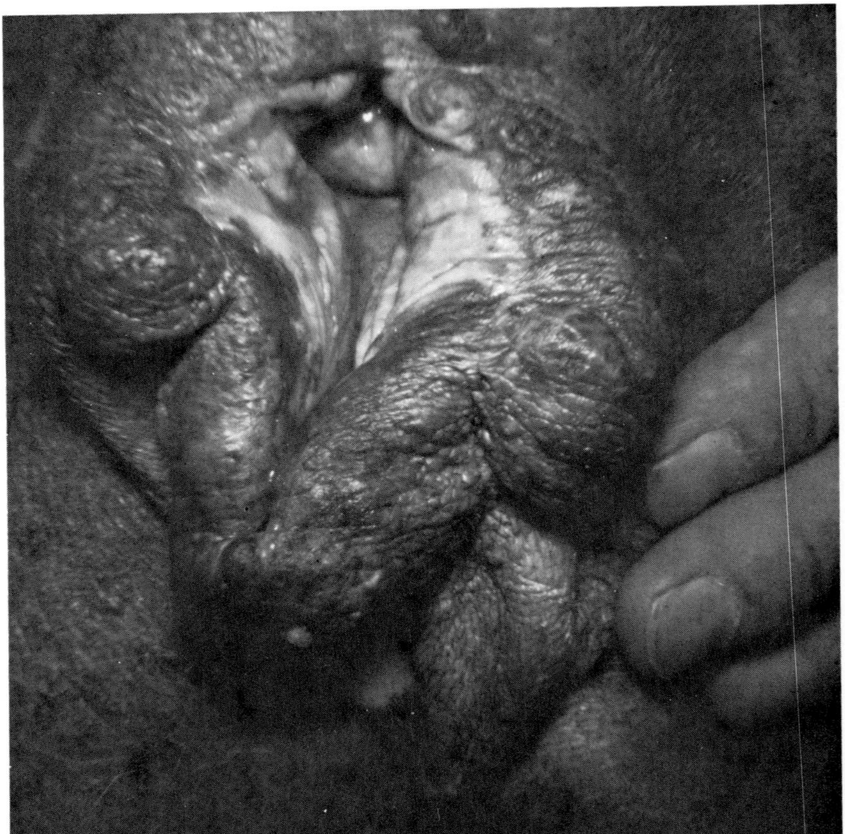

Fig. 11–4. Enlarged and swollen vulva of a seven-year-old collie dog with a functional granulosa-theca cell tumor of the ovary.

metestrus and in the first part of pregnancy. While the corpora lutea mainly secrete progesterone, estrogens and some intermediary androgens are also produced. The hilar cells differ from the rest of the stroma in that they resemble cells of testicular origin and probably secrete androgens.

Hormone-producing ovarian tumors are rare in the dog. The most common mesenchymal tumor is the granulosa-theca cell tumor. The cells resemble those found in the graafian follicle, and the composition may vary from completely granulosal to completely thecal. Generally the two cell types are mixed, but one or the other tissue usually predominates. These tumors may or may not be functional, but when they are, they are usually estrogen secreting, and the affected bitch shows evidence of estrogenic stimulation. The vulva is greatly swollen, similar to a dog in estrus with maximal estrogen stimulation (Fig. 11–4). This estrogenic effect results in attraction of

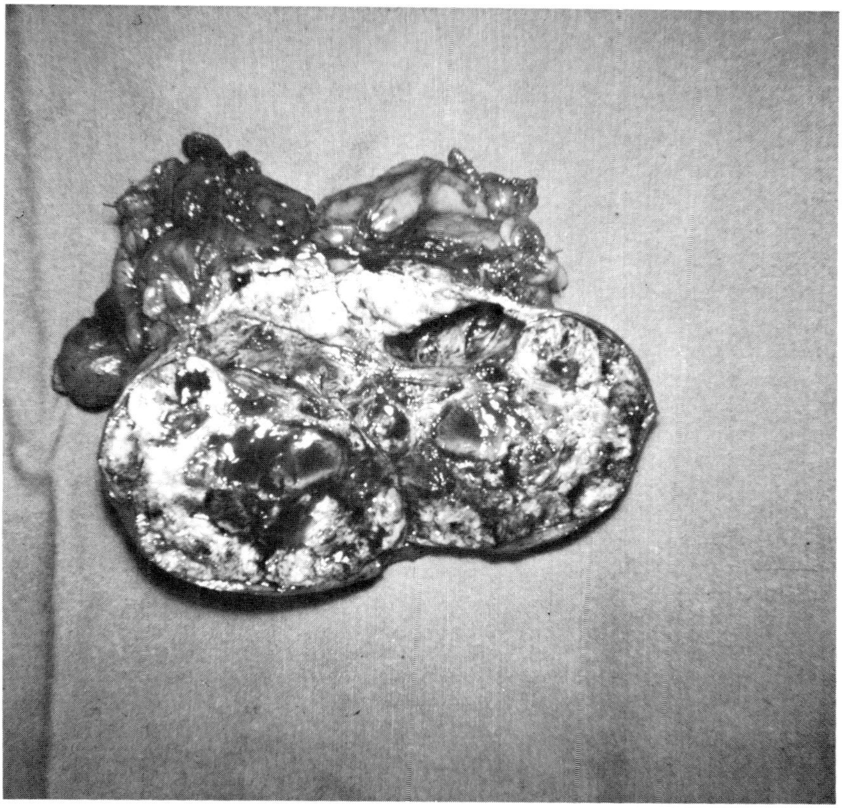

Fig. 11–5. Cut section of the ovarian granulosa-theca cell tumor removed from the dog shown in Fig. 11–4.

male dogs, vulvar swelling, and vaginal discharge progressing over a period of time. In gross appearance, granulosa-theca cell tumors may be solid to partly cystic, and vary in color from grayish to yellow. Consistency is usually firm, but large tumors may contain areas of cystic degeneration (Fig. 11–5). Histologic appearance of the granulosa-theca cell tumor does not reflect hormonal activity. At times granulosa-theca cell tumors undergo what appears to be typical luteinization, which may affect all or part of the tumor. In the past, such tumors were called luteomas.

The arrhenoblastoma is a tumor that appears to be composed of cells resembling the Leydig cells of the testes. This tumor is rare in the dog. In man this tumor is typically virilizing or masculinizing when functional.

The terminology for many ovarian tumors varies widely. Most are rare, and the functional nature is equally rare. With the exception of the granulosa-theca cell tumor, the ovarian tumors are only a clinical curiosity.

PHARMACOLOGIC ESTRUS INHIBITION

It is desirable to be able to inhibit estrus in the pet dog. Ovariohysterectomy is satisfactory for some pet owners, but its permanence is not desirable for owners that want to breed the animal at a later time.

Estrus control in the dog offers some different problems from fertility control in people. Certain steroidal compounds (the Pill) are successful in inhibiting ovulation and conception in women. In the dog, the problem is somewhat different. The mechanisms to be inhibited are estrus and the attraction of male dogs. It is not important whether ovulation itself is inhibited, as long as the external signs of estrus are prevented.

Various steroids have been used in an attempt to control the estrous cycle in the bitch. Most of these drugs have been either progestational or androgenic compounds. Although earlier studies suggested that exogenous progestational compounds could result in endometrial cystic hyperplasia-pyometra, this factor did not distract a number of drug companies and other investigators from using other progestogens in the dog. Some of these compounds are effective in inhibiting estrus in the bitch, but are controversial because of their effect on the canine endometrium. One long-acting compound, medroxyprogesterone acetate (Promone), given subcutaneously, can suppress estrus from 6 to 26.5 months. However, clinicians in the field report that repeated use increases incidence of endometrial cystic hyperplasia-pyometra. Reevaluation of this compound showed a 20.9% incidence of endometrial stimulation in treated bitches.

It has also been shown that medroxyprogesterone acetate does not result in endometrial hyperplasia in the ovariectomized bitch, demonstrating that the ovary and/or its secretion must be present for this progestogen to affect the endometrium. Probably the contribution of estrogen secretion from the ovary is synergistic with the progestogen in producing the endometrial hyperplasia. The actual incidence of pyometra in one controlled experiment of dogs on medroxyprogesterone acetate was only 2.8%, but the same study indicated that the frequency of all uterine disorders, such as pyometra, endometritis, and metritis, was actually 9.9%. This high rate of uterine abnormality makes this compound unacceptable for estrus control in the dog.

Another progestogen, megestrol acetate (Ovaban), has been reported effective for estrus control in the dog. This compound is administered orally. The manufacturers claim that the drug is well tolerated, and that confirmed cases of pyometra are less than 1%. However, this drug has not been critically evaluated by the veterinary profession in general. Further experience with this progestogen is necessary before the drug has general acceptance.

Since the problem in the dog is to control estrus and the attraction of male dogs, different types of compounds may be found effective. Antiestrogenic compounds need to be investigated inasmuch as these compounds can block the effect of estrogens at the target or peripheral tissue level, and may not produce the undesirable side effects, seen with the progestational compounds.

PHYSIOLOGY OF THE MALE DOG

The canine testes are normally scrotal at birth. Occasionally in some breeds or families within a breed, the testes may descend into the scrotum after birth. In some cases the testes do not become scrotal until seven or eight months of age. For testes to be functional and reproductive, they must become scrotal before puberty.

The canine testes secrete androgens, i.e., testosterone, dihydrotestosterone, and androstenedione. The androgens affect the general morphology of the developing male with increased muscle development, and are also involved in the development of the male micturition pattern. Androgens are also necessary for normal development of the secondary sex tissues. The os penis appears to depend on adequate amounts of androgens, as well as growth hormone, for normal size and calcification. Normally the os penis calcifies at four to five months of age.

Castration of the immature dog prevents development of the male micturition pattern of lifting the leg. However, administration of exogenous androgens to the castrated dog reestablishes this pattern. Similarly, androgen administration to female puppies and spayed bitches produces the male micturition pattern. One study has shown that local anesthesia of the olfactory epithelium in the male dog causes a disappearance of the male micturition pattern, which is replaced by the female pattern. When anesthesia wears off, the male pattern reappears. The results of this experiment suggest that this reflex depends on an intact olfactory epithelium. It raises the possibility that pheromones may be important in reinforcing this pattern of behavior.

Testosterone, dihydrotestosterone, and androstenedione have been isolated in spermatic vein blood of the dog. The catabolism of testosterone in the dog is different from that in man. Approximately 20% of injected testosterone is excreted within 48 hours in canine urine. The specific catabolites have not been identified, but testosterone is not metabolized to 17-ketosteroids as in man.

The androgens also affect the prostate gland. Castration results in atrophy of the prostate gland, but testosterone administration to the castrated dog prevents such atrophy. Large amounts of androgens experimentally produce prostatic hypertrophy in the dog; this action can be blocked by the antiandrogen, cyproterone acetate.

Castrating the male dog before puberty abolishes sexual behavior. However, if castration is not carried out until after sexual maturity, the decrease in the sexual behavior is less complete. Sexual performance declines progressively following castration in the sexually mature dog, but some dogs remain vigorous sexually for as long as two years postoperatively. Sexual behavior after castration is not due to a compensatory increase in adrenal androgens, since adrenalectomy following castration does not alter the response to castration. In man, approximately one third of the total androgens are of testicular origin in the male, whereas two thirds are of adrenal origin. The specific contribution of these two glands to the androgen production in the dog is not established.

Some clinicians have suggested that insufficient androgens produce an abnormality in the dog's skin and haircoat. However, castrated and adrenalectomized dogs without any sex hormone supplementation continue to have normal skin and haircoats.

HYPOFUNCTION OF THE TESTES

Information concerning the etiology of infertility in the male dog is practically nonexistent as are satisfactory methods of therapy. Even if complicated and expensive endocrine assays were available and used for evaluating male dogs, these assays would show that most infertile male dogs have no treatable disease. Because of the disappointing results of therapy seen in the clinic, many clinicians have abandoned any type of complicated investigation; instead they fall into the easy habit of using empirical medication, such as thyroid supplementation, low doses of testosterone, vitamin and mineral supplementation, knowing that these medications do not improve the patient's fertility.

With primary hypogonadism the testes do not develop at puberty, but remain small and immature. Occasionally these dogs respond to the administration of chorionic gonadotropin; therefore, some cases appear to result from an insufficiency of endogenous gonadotropin secretion.

Secondary hypofunction of the testes in the male dog results from suppression of testicular function due to abnormalities originating outside the testes after testicular development. Hypothyroidism decreases fertility in the male dog, specifically decreasing sperm count and possibly lowering libido. In canine Cushing's syndrome the high level of serum cortisol suppresses gonadotropin secretion, with both decreased sperm count and testicular atrophy occurring in about 30% of the cases.

In cases of hypogonadism associated with diseases of other endocrine tissues, correction of the primary disorder often results in correction of the infertility. However, in many cases of infertility in the male dog, the cause is not evident.

CRYPTORCHIDISM

The spermatic tubules in both the cryptorchid and normal testis grow at the same rate early in life. However, with advancing age and before puberty, the tubules of the properly descended testis begin to increase substantially in diameter, while the tubules of the cryptorchid testis decrease in size. This difference has led to the conclusion that, if the cryptorchid testes remain outside the scrotum after a specific age (somewhere around the time of puberty), they will suffer definite and permanent damage. Correction of cryptorchidism must occur before sexual maturity if the male is to have fertile testes.

Whenever extrascrotal testes are present, it is necessary to determine whether true cryptorchidism or a retracted testis is present. The retracted testis has a cremasteric reflex that is active in pulling the testis into a high position. Often, with increasing age this reflex becomes less active, and the testis is permitted to be spontaneously lowered to the scrotum. The retracted testis in the inguinal canal can be pushed gently down into the scrotum. In true cryptorchidism, the testis cannot be felt or, if palpable, cannot be pushed down into the scrotal sac. The retracted testis usually is not a problem, since most of these descend without any medical interference.

Over the years medical treatment of cryptorchidism in man has been a controversial topic. Some clinicians in the past reported success with one of two types of hormonal therapy, either administration of gonadotropins or treatment with androgens. However, in recent years some controlled studies do not substantiate the success of hormonal therapy. Successful results following hormonal therapy may have been achieved in children who had retracted testes that would have come down spontaneously in subsequent years. Many believe that surgical correction of this disorder in man is preferable. Surgical correction or orchiopexy must be done before puberty. The preferable age for the surgical operation is debatable, but generally it is carried out between the ages of four to nine years of age in man.

Surgical correction of cryptorchidism in the dog is not recommended for a number of reasons. This type of surgical procedure disqualifies the animal for American Kennel Club registration. Based on limited data, it appears that some cases of cryptorchidism in the dog are hereditary. Therefore, veterinarians usually recommend that the cryptorchid dog not be used in a breeding program in which the defect of cryptorchidism will become established in the particular line. Although it is not always possible to determine whether the particular affected animal is carrying a hereditary defect, the possibility often precludes using the cryptorchid dog for breeding purposes.

In dog and man, if a testis remains extrascrotal after puberty, the incidence of testicular tumors increases in this cryptorchid testis. The incidence of tumors increases with age, so it is recommended that cryptorchid testes be removed early in the animal's life. I recommend that cryptorchid testes be removed between one and two years of age.

TESTICULAR TUMORS

Testicular tumors are relatively common in the dog. Most of these tumors can be essentially classified into one of three types: the Sertoli cell tumor (sustentacular cell tumor, tubular adenoma), the interstitial cell tumor (Leydig's cell tumor), or the seminoma (spermatogonioma). The embryonal carcinoma, chorionepithelioma, or teratoma are rare in the dog.

The **interstitial cell tumor** is the most common testicular tumor in the dog. These tumors are small, often ranging from 1 to 9 centimeters in diameter. In gross appearance, they are raised, discrete, and yellowish or brownish (Fig. 11–6). Histologically these tumors are composed of enlarged Leydig's cells, which are arranged diffusely and supported by a delicate vascular framework (Figs. 11–7 and 11–8). When these tumors are functional in man, they are usually androgen secreting. When present in children, they cause precocious puberty development. In the dog these tumors do not appear to have functional significance. Since these tumors are seen mainly in the sexually mature dog, if androgen secreting, the excess androgens would not be evident.

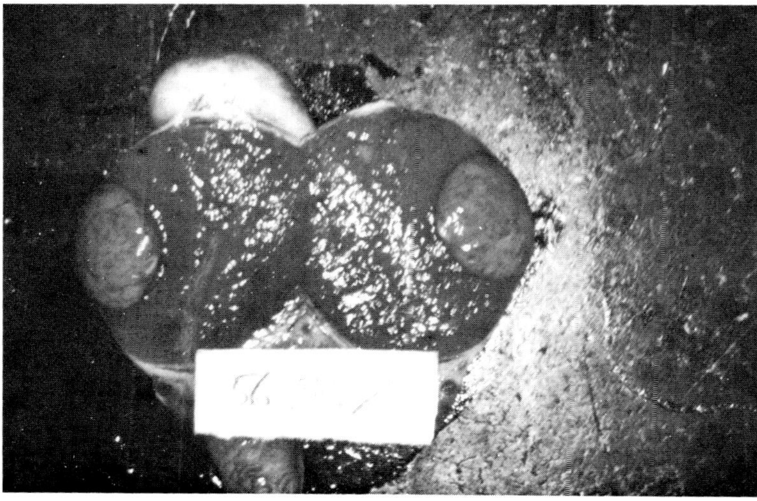

Fig. 11–6. Cut section of a testis with an interstitial cell tumor.

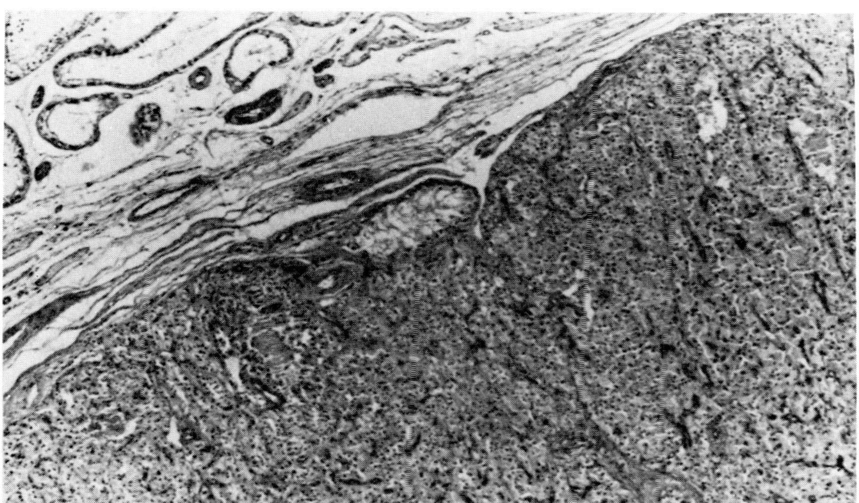

Fig. 11–7. Interstitial cell tumor of the testis ×34. This tumor contains Leydig's cells, which are arranged diffusely and supported by a delicate vascular framework. (Courtesy John T. McGrath, University of Pennsylvania.)

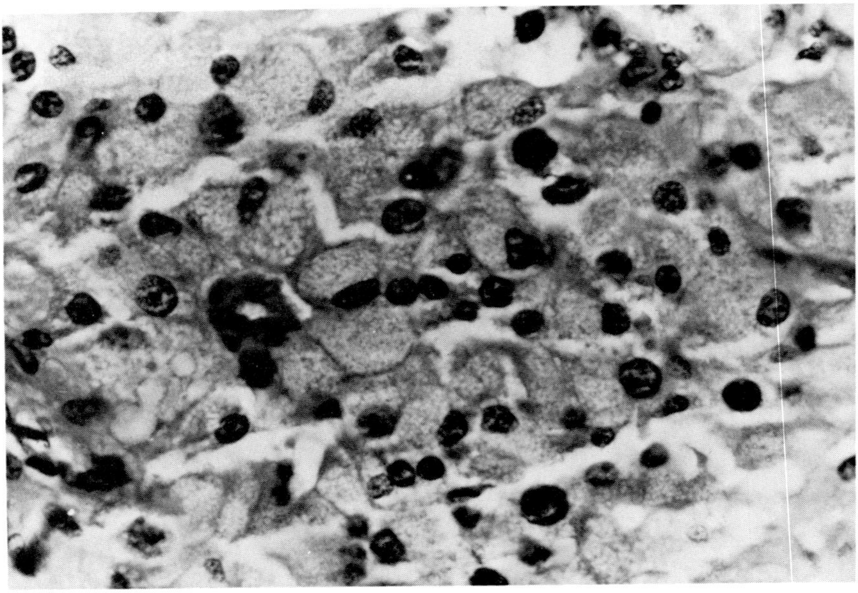

Fig. 11–8. Interstitial cell tumor of the testis ×289. A higher magnification of the tumor shown in Fig. 11–7. (Courtesy John T. McGrath, University of Pennsylvania.)

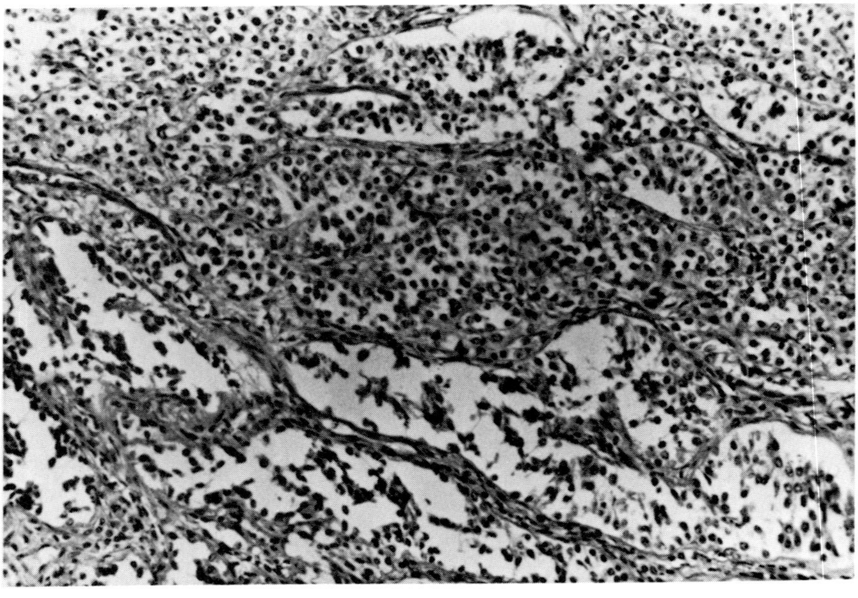

Fig. 11–9. Sertoli cell adenoma of the testis. This tumor contains sheet-like masses of elongated Sertoli cells arranged in a somewhat glandular pattern. (Courtesy John T. McGrath, University of Pennsylvania.)

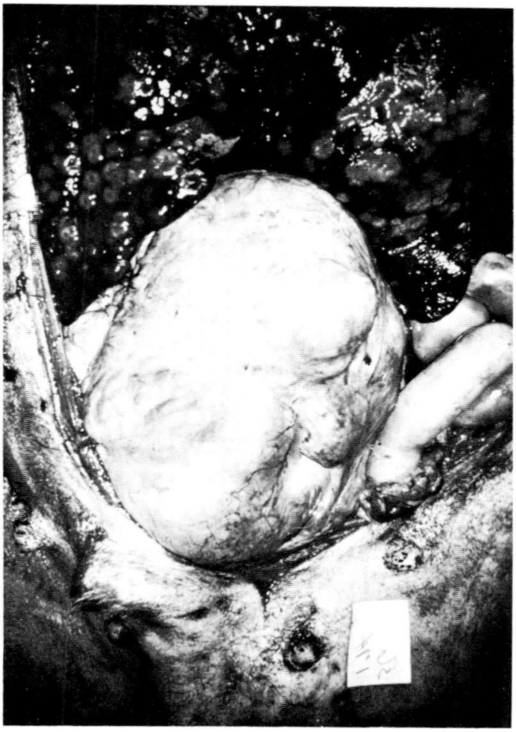

Fig. 11–10. Sertoli cell adenocarcinoma. Primary tumor originated in the retained testis (center). Multiple metastases are present in the liver (above).

The **Sertoli cell tumors** are interesting because they are frequently associated with feminization. The feminized dog attracts other male dogs, and thus simulates a bitch during estrus. The dogs also exhibit loss of libido, gynecomastia, and atrophy of the unaffected testis. Normal growth or replacement of hair ceases, and symmetrical alopecia appears at the site of maximal abrasion or wear. Clinical signs vary in their degree of severity; often only signs of gynecomastia, alopecia, or attraction to other male dogs are evident.

The Sertoli cell tumors have a higher degree of functional behavior when the testis is extrascrotal. In addition, the functional nature of the tumor appears to depend on the relative size of the tumor; the larger the tumor, usually the more pronounced the clinical signs. Occasionally small, pea-sized tumors may be functional. Bioassay techniques have shown that these tumors are estrogen-secreting. However, recent studies have not been able to demonstrate an elevation in the usual estrogens, such as estradiol-17β, estradiol-17α, or estrone. It has been suggested that the feminization is the result of estrogenic material of unknown structure.

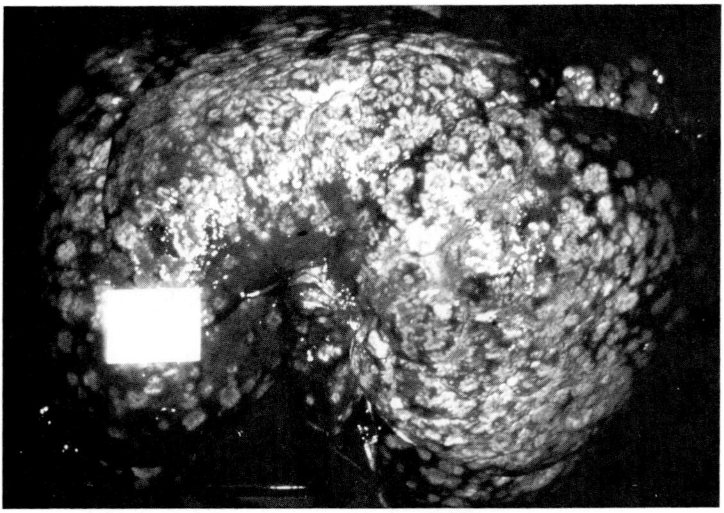

Fig. 11–11. Metastatic Sertoli cell adenocarcinoma in the liver (removed at necropsy from case shown in Fig. 11–10).

Histologically the Sertoli cell tumors may appear benign or malignant (Fig. 11–9). In general the small tumors have a benign microscopic appearance, while the larger ones usually have more malignant characteristics. Biologically metastases are rarely seen. With functional tumors in which the primary mass has been removed, feminization may recur. If so, it indicates the formation of new functional metastatic lesions (Figs. 11–10 and 11–11).

The **seminoma** is derived from the seminiferous tubules. These tumors are not functional in the dog. Their histologic appearance may be deceiving; on occasion they appear to be malignant. Metastasis of seminomas in the dog is relatively infrequent.

HERMAPHRODITISM AND PSEUDOHERMAPHRODITISM

The classification of intersexes may be extensive because of the variables of chromosomal pattern, gonadal sexual tissue, internal accessory reproductive structures, and external genital morphology. Classically, the true **hermaphrodite** possesses both ovarian and testicular tissue. Each gonad may be an ovotestis, or a testicle may appear on one side and an ovary on the other. Occasionally the individual has two ovaries or two testes. The appearance of the external genitals ranges from near-female to normal male. The chromosomal pattern may be male or female, irrespective of other sexual structures.

Ambiguous-looking external genitalia are encountered in some varieties of hermaphroditism; i.e., the external genitalia remain incompletely differentiated as either male or female. Ambiguous external genitalia are always unfinished genitalia. It is embryologically impossible for a hermaphrodite to possess two full sets of external organs, one male and one female. Intersexuality or hermaphroditism is an anomaly of embryologic and fetal sexual differentiation. The external genitalia of both male and female are homologous and differentiate from the same anlagen. The internal reproductive structures, by contrast, do not differentiate from the same anlagen. In this respect, the embryo is initially hermaphroditic, possessing both wolffian ducts of the male and müllerian ducts of the female. Subsequently, one set of ducts proliferates while the other atrophies.

Experimentally it has been shown that, with mammalian sexual differentiation, female development takes precedence over sexual differentiation as a male. When male rabbit embryos were castrated at

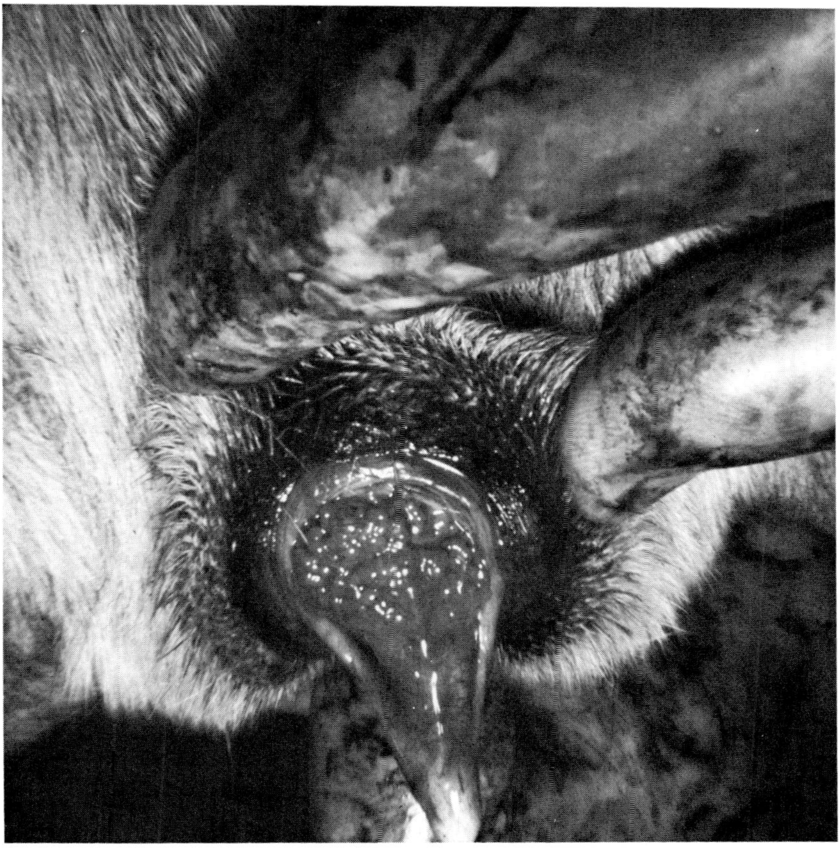

Fig. 11–12. Enlarged clitoris in a male pseudohermaphrodite.

a critical time during gestation, the embryos developed anatomically as females. However, when castration is carried out only a few days later, it can no longer suppress the male differentiation. Based on these classical experiments, it appears that the developing testes and the secretion of androgens are necessary for the full development of male genitalia. It has also been shown that unilateral castration of the male embryo produces female differentiation only on the castrated side.

Apparently the counterpart intersex of this type of in utero castration would be the **male pseudohermaphrodite,** which develops in some cases of testicular hypoplasia. Classically the individual that has testes with either ambiguous or female external genitalia is called a **male pseudohermaphrodite.** This type of pseudohermaphroditism is

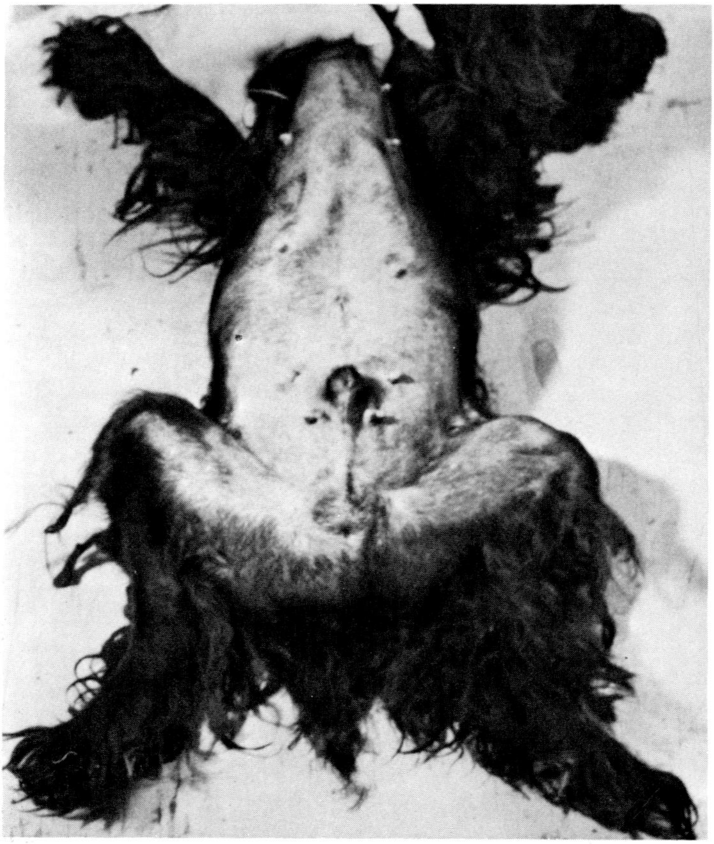

Fig. 11–13. External genitalia of a female pseudohermaphrodite cocker spaniel. (From McFeely, R. A., and Biggers, J. D.: Vet. Rec., 77:696, 1965.)

the most common intersex seen in the canine species. The gonads are usually retained testes, and may be somewhat functional if any masculinization exists in an otherwise feminine genital tract. The enlargement of the clitoris is the most common manifestation of the rudimentary androgen secretion from the hypoplastic gonad (Fig. 11–12).

In another type of male pseudohermaphroditism, the etiology is less than perfectly understood. This type has male sex chromosome patterns and a well-developed uterus and tubes coexistent with testes that, instead of being aplastic or vestigial, are well differentiated and near normal in size. The external genitalia may not be completely feminized; occasionally a rudimentary penis and scrotum may be formed. This intersex often has some degree of hypospadias present.

Female pseudohermaphrodites are genetic females with varying degrees of masculinization of the external genitalia (Fig. 11–13). In man this disorder is most commonly due to congenital adrenal hyperplasia, a disorder characterized by enzymatic defects and insufficiencies of the adrenal cortex, which result in the overproduction of some androgenic substances. This type of disorder has not been recognized in the dog.

Female pseudohermaphroditism may also be the result of excess androgens produced abnormally during pregnancy, or it can result from exogenous administration of various steroids during the early part of pregnancy. In the former situation, ovarian or adrenocortical tumors producing excessive androgens are a possible cause of this type of induced female pseudohermaphroditism. According to some reports, androgens or progestational compounds have masculinized the female pups during pregnancy. In this situation, progesterone is readily converted to androgens, resulting in the development of female pseudohermaphroditism.

SELECTED READING

The Ovary

1. Andersen, A. C.: Granulosa-cell tumor in a beagle. J. Am. Vet. Med. Assoc., *143*:384, 1963.
2. Anderson, R. K., Gilmore, C. E., and Schnelle, G. B.: Utero-ovarian disorders associated with use of medroxyprogesterone in dogs. J. Am. Vet. Med. Assoc., *146*:1311, 1965.
3. Bachelor, A., Bell, E. T., and Christie, D. W.: Urinary oestrogen levels in the beagle bitch. J. Endocrinol., *51*:26, 1971.
4. Barclay, D. L., and Sternberg, W. H.: A classification of intersexes. South. Med. J., *59*:1383, 1966.
5. Barnawell, E. B.: Analysis of the direct action of prolactin and steroids on mammary tissue of the dog in organ culture. Endocrinology, *80*:1083, 1967.
6. Bell, E. T., Parkes, M. F., and Christie, D. W.: Gonadotrophin excretion in ovariectomized bitches. J. Reprod. Fertil., *27*:83, 1971.
7. Bell, E. T., and Christie, D. W.: Erythrocytes and leucocytes in the vaginal smear of the beagle bitch. Vet. Rec., *88*:546, 1971.

8. Bell, E. T, Christie, D. W., and Younglai, E. V.: Plasma oestrogen levels during the canine oestrous cycle. J. Endocrinol., *51*:225, 1971.
9. Bleicher, N.: Behavior of the bitch during parturition. J. Am. Vet. Med. Assoc., *140*:1076, 1962.
10. Brodey, R. S., and Fidler, I. J.: Clinical and pathologic findings in bitches treated with progestational compounds. J. Am. Vet. Med. Assoc., *149*:1406, 1966.
11. Brodey, R. S., and Roszel, J. F.: Neoplasms of the canine uterus, vagina, and vulva: a clinicopathologic survey of 90 cases. J. Am. Vet. Med. Assoc., *151*:1294, 1967.
12. Bryan, H. S.: Parenteral use of medroxyprogesterone acetate as an antifertility agent in the bitch. Am. J. Vet. Res., *34*:659, 1973.
13. Burke, T. J., and Reynolds, H. A., Jr.: Megestrol acetate for estrus postponement in the bitch. J. Am. Vet. Med. Assoc., *167*:285, 1975.
14. Christie, D. W., et al.: Peripheral plasma progesterone levels during the canine oestrous cycle. Acta Endocrinol., *68*:543, 1971.
15. Cotchin, E.: Spontaneous uterine cancer in animals. Br. J. Cancer, *18*:209, 1964.
16. Curtis, E. M., and Grant, R. P.: Masculinization of female pups by progestogens. J. Am. Vet. Med. Assoc., *144*:395, 1964.
17. Del Campo, C. H., and Ginther, O. J.: Arteries and veins of uterus and ovaries in dogs and cats. Am. J. Vet. Res., *35*:409, 1974.
18. Dow, C.: The cystic hyperplasia-pyometra complex in the bitch. J. Comp. Pathol. Ther., *69*:237, 1959.
19. Edqvist, L. E., et al.: Blood plasma levels of progesterone and oestradiol in the dog during the oestrous cycle and pregnancy. Acta Endocrinol., *78*:554, 1975.
20. Eik-Nes, K. B.: Comparative endocrinology of reproduction. Gen. Comp. Endocrinol., [Suppl.] *2*:87, 1969.
21. Fidler, I. J., et al.: Relationship of estrous irregularity, pseudopregnancy, and pregnancy to canine pyometra. J. Am. Vet. Med. Assoc., *149*:1043, 1966.
22. Fitch, K. L.: A study of uterine glycogen during the estrous cycle of the dog. J. Morphol., *113*:331, 1963.
23. Fowler, E. H., Loeb, W. F., and Wilson, G. P.: Vaginal cytologic examination of intact and ovariohysterectomized bitches with mammary neoplasia. Am. J. Vet. Res., *31*:51, 1970.
24. Gier, H. T.: Estrous Cycle in the Bitch: Vaginal Fluids. *In* Veterinary Scope, Vol. 2. Upjohn Company, Kalamazoo, 1960, p. 2.
25. Gill, H. P., et al.: Artificial insemination of beagle bitches with freshly collected, liquid-stored, and frozen-stored semen. Am. J. Vet. Res., *31*:1807, 1970.
26. Hadley, J. C.: Unconjugated oestrogen and progesterone concentrations in the blood of bitches with false pregnancy and pyometra. Vet. Rec., *96*:545, 1975.
27. Hill, R., and Dumas, K.: The use of dogs for studies of toxicity of contraceptive hormones. Meeting on Pharmacological Models to Assess Toxicity and Side Effects of Fertility Regulating Agents, Geneva, Switzerland, 1973, Syntex Corporation, Palo Alto, CA.
28. Holst, P. A., and Phemister, R. D.: The prenatal development of the dog: preimplantation events. Biol. Reprod., *5*:194, 1971.
29. Holst, P. A., and Phemister, R. D.: Onset of diestrus in the beagle bitch: definition and significance. Am. J. Vet. Res., *35*:401, 1974.
30. Holst, P. A., and Phemister, R. D.: Temporal sequence of events in the estrous cycle of the bitch. Am. J. Vet. Res., *36*:705, 1975.
31. Jones, G. E., et al.: Plasma oestradiol, luteinizing hormone and progesterone during the oestrous cycle in the beagle bitch. J. Endocrinol., *57*:331, 1973.
32. Marshall, F. H. A., and Jolly, W. A.: Contributions to the physiology of mammalian reproduction. Part I. The oestrous cycle in the dog. Part II. The ovary as an organ of internal secretion. Philos. Trans. R. Soc. Lond., ser. B, *198*:99, 1905.
33. McFeeley, R. A., and Biggers, J. D.: A rare case of female pseudohermaphroditism in the dog. Vet. Rec., *77*:696, 1965.
34. Metzler, F., Jr., Eleftheriou, B. E., and Fox, M.: Free estrogens in dog plasma during the estrous cycle and pregnancy. Proc. Soc. Exp. Biol. Med., *121*:374, 1966.
35. Newberne, J. W., Kuhn, W. L., and Elsea, J. R.: Toxicologic studies on clomiphene. Toxicol. Applied Pharmacol., *9*:44, 1966.

36. Norris, H. J., Garner, F. M., and Taylor, H. B.: Comparative pathology of ovarian neoplasms. J. Comp. Pathol., *80*:399, 1970.
37. Phemister, R. D., et al.: Time of ovulation in the beagle bitch. Biol. Reprod., *8*:74, 1973.
38. Roszel, J. F.: Genital Cytology of the Bitch. *In* Veterinary Scope, Vol. 19. The Upjohn Corporation, Kalamazoo, 1975, p. 3.
39. Schutt, A. J., and Hayles, A. B.: Intersex. Mayo Clin. Proc., *39*:363, 1964.
40. Simmons, J. G., and Hamner, C. E.: Inhibition of estrus in the dog with testosterone implants. Am. J. Vet. Res., *34*:1409, 1973.
41. Smith, M. S., and McDonald, L. E.: Serum levels of luteinizing hormone and progesterone during the estrous cycle, pseudopregnancy and pregnancy in the dog. Endocrinology, *94*:404, 1974.
42. Sokolowski, J. H.: Reproductive features and patterns in the bitch. J. Am. Anim. Hosp. Assoc., *9*:71, 1973.
43. Sokolowski, J. H., Zimbelman, R. G., and Goyings, L. S.: Canine reproduction: reproductive organs and related structures of the nonparous, parous, and postpartum bitch. Am. J. Vet. Res., *34*:1001, 1973.
44. Sokolowski, J. H., and Zimbelman, R. G. Canine reproduction: effects of a single injection of medroxyprogesterone acetate on the reproductive organs of intact and ovariectomized bitches. Am. J. Vet. Res., *34*:1501, 1973.
45. Sokolowski, J. H., and Zimbelman, R. G.: Canine reproduction: effects of a single injection of medroxyprogesterone acetate on the reproductive organs of the bitch. Am. J. Vet. Res., *34*:1493, 1973.
46. Sokolowski, J. H., and Zimbelman, R. G.: Canine reproduction: effects of multiple treatments of medroxyprogesterone acetate on reproductive organs of the bitch. Am. J. Vet. Res., *35*:1285, 1974.
47. Taylor, G. P.: Pill produces puppies. Kennel Rev., *72*:104, 1970.
48. Verma, O. P., and Chibuzo, G. A.: Hormonal influences on motility of canine uterine horns. Am. J. Vet. Res., *35*:23, 1974.
49. Wilkinson, G. T.: The treatment of mammary tumours in the bitch and a comparison with the cat. Vet. Rec., *89*:13, 1971.

The Testes

1. Brodey, R. S., and Martin, J. E.: Sertoli cell neoplasms in the dog. J. Am. Vet. Med. Assoc., *133*:249, 1958.
2. Brown, R. C., Swanton, M. C., and Brinkhous, K. M.: Canine hemophilia and male pseudohermaphroditism. Lab. Invest., *12*:961, 1963.
3. Clough, E., et al.: An XXY sex-chromosome constitution in a dog with testicular hypoplasia and congenital heart disease. Cytogenetics, *9*:71, 1970.
4. Coffin, D. L., Munson, T. O., and Scully, R. E.: Functional Sertoli cell tumor with metastasis in a dog. J. Am. Vet. Med. Assoc., *121*:352, 1952.
5. Comhaire, F., Mattheeuws, D., and Vermeulen, A.: Testosterone and oestradiol in dogs with testicular tumours. Acta Endocrinol., 77:408, 1974.
6. Cotchin, E.: Testicular neoplasms in dogs. J. Comp. Pathol. Ther., *70*:232, 1960.
7. Dain, A. R.: Intersexuality in a cocker spaniel dog. J. Reprod. Fertil., *39*:365, 1974.
8. Dow, C.: Testicular tumours in the dog. J. Comp. Pathol., *72*:247, 1962.
9. Edols, J. H., and Allan, G. S.: A case of male pseudohermaphroditism in a cocker spaniel. Aust. Vet. J., *44*:287, 1968.
10. Ehrlich, R. M., et al.: Effect of gonadotropin in cryptorchism. J. Urol., *102*:793, 1969.
11. Eik-Nes, K. B.: Secretion of testosterone in anesthetized dogs. Endocrinology, *71*:101, 1962.
12. Eleftheriou, B. E., and Stanley, W. C.: Influence of testosterone propionate and growth hormone on the os penis in the dog. Endocrinology, *72*:161, 1963.
13. Frey, D. C., Tyler, D. E., and Ramsey, F. K.: Pyometra associated with bilateral cryptorchism and Sertoli's cell tumor in a male pseudohermaphroditic dog. J. Am. Vet. Med. Assoc., *146*:723, 1965.
14. Gross, R. E., and Replogle, R. L.: Treatment of the undescended testis. Postgrad. Med., *34*:266, 1963.

15. Haltmeyer, G. C., and Eik-Nes, K. B.: Transport of 5α-dihydrotestosterone by testicular lymph in the dog. J. Reprod. Fertil., *36*:41, 1974.
16. Hartig, P. R.: The problem of male infertility. Lancet, *83*:307, 1963.
17. Huggins, C., and Pazos, R., Jr.: Studies on tumors of the testis. II. The morphology of testicular tumors of dogs. Am. J. Pathol., *21*:299, 1945.
18. Jones, H. W., Jr., and Zourlas, P. A.: Clinical, histologic and cytogenetic findings in male hermaphroditism. Obstet. Gynecol., *25*:597, 1965.
19. Kelch, R. P., et al.: Estradiol and testosterone secretion by human, simian, and canine testes, in males with hypogonadism and in male pseudohermaphrodites with the feminizing testes syndrome. J. Clin. Invest., *51*:824, 1972.
20. Lipowitz, A. J., et al.: Testicular neoplasms and concomitant clinical changes in the dog. J. Am. Vet. Med. Assoc., *163*:1364, 1973.
21. Merrill, J. A., and Ramsey, J. E.: True hermaphroditism. Obstet. Gynecol., *22*:505, 1963.
22. Mostofi, F. K.: Testicular tumors. Cancer, *32*:1186, 1973.
23. Oh, R., and Tamaoki, B.: In vitro biosynthesis of androgens in canine testes. Acta Endocrinol., *74*:615, 1973.
24. Pierrepoint, C. G., et al.: Steroid metabolism of a Sertoli cell tumour of the testis of a dog with feminization and alopecia and of the normal canine testis. J. Endocrinol., *38*:61, 1967.
25. Pierrepoint, C. G.: The metabolism in vitro of dehydroepiandrosterone and dehydroepiandrosterone sulphate by Sertoli cell tumours of the testis of two dogs with clinical signs of hyperoestrogenism. J. Endocrinol., *42*:99, 1968.
26. Potter, W. R., and Riggott, J. M.: A pseudohermaphrodite dog. Vet. Rec., *80*:647, 1967.
27. Reif, J. S., and Brodey, R. S.: The relationship between cryptorchidism and canine testicular neoplasia. J. Am. Vet. Med. Assoc., *155*:2005, 1969.
28. Schultz, M. G.: Male pseudohermaphroditism diagnosed with aid of sex chromatin technique. J. Am. Vet. Med. Assoc., *140*:241, 1962.
29. Scully, R. E., and Coffin, D. L.: Canine testicular tumors. Cancer, *5*:592, 1952.
30. Siegel, E. T., et al.: Conversion of 6,7-H^3-estradiol-17β into estrone and estradiol-17α in the mature male dog. Proc. Soc. Exp. Biol. Med., *8*:533, 1962.
31. Siegel, E. T., and Dorfman, R. I.: A chemical method for the determination of estrone, 17α-estradiol and 17β-estradiol in canine urine. Steroids, *1*:409, 1963.
32. Siegel, E. T., et al.: An estrogen study in the feminized dog with testicular neoplasia. Endocrinology, *80*:272, 1967.
33. Smith, A. M., Lattimer, J. K., and Rezvan, M.: Current therapy for undescended testicle. N. Y. State J. Med., *73*:2557, 1973.
34. Streett, C. S.: Sertoli-cell carcinoma and multiple metastasis in a dog. Cornell Vet., *57*:597, 1967.
35. Vermeulen, A., and Verdonck, L.: Some studies on the biological significance of free testosterone. J. Steroid Biochem., *3*:421, 1972.
36. Wachstein, M., and Scorza, A.: Male pseudohermaphroditism. Am. J. Clin. Pathol., *21*:10, 1951.

Index

Page numbers in *italics* indicate illustrations.